REWORDING THE BRAIN

Legendary crossword-maker in *The Age* and *The Sydney Morning Herald*, as well as Wordplay columnist with 'Spectrum', David Astle is a full-time word nerd. He is also a prolific author and broadcaster, and an ambassador for Dementia Australia.

DAVID ASTLE

REWORDING THE BRAIN

How cryptic crosswords can improve your memory
and boost the power and agility of your brain

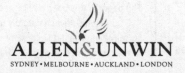

ALLEN&UNWIN
SYDNEY · MELBOURNE · AUCKLAND · LONDON

To Heather and Barry, the carer and the cared

This edition published in 2020
First published in 2018

Allen & Unwin
83 Alexander Street
Crows Nest NSW 2065
Australia
Phone: (61 2) 8425 0100
Email: info@allenandunwin.com
Web: www.allenandunwin.com

A catalogue record for this
book is available from the
National Library of Australia

ISBN 978 1 76087 694 4

Internal design by Bookhouse
Set in Adobe Caslon Pro by Bookhouse, Sydney
Printed in Australia by McPherson's Printing Group

10 9 8 7 6 5 4 3 2 1

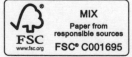

The paper in this book is FSC® certified.
FSC® promotes environmentally responsible,
socially beneficial and economically viable
management of the world's forests.

'The essence of the independent mind lies not in what it thinks, but in how it thinks.'

Christopher Hitchens

CONTENTS

THE EXPERIMENT

'Have you ever been shot?' asks the nurse.

'No.'

'Tattoos?'

'No.'

She ticks a box. 'Prosthetic limb? Internal staples? Plates? Hip replacement?'

'No. No. No. And again, no.'

She ticks away. As does my countdown clock on the wall. In a few minutes, for the first time in history, a human brain will solve a cryptic crossword while being scanned inside a giant tube. My brain, to be precise. I'm nervous as a kitten—speaking as the guinea pig.

Renee, the nurse, continues with her questions, working her pen down the list, from allergies to phobias, from dentures to nicotine patches, as I keep my eye on the clock. What comes next, the whole experiment in the tube next door, is one big risk. Less for reasons of safety than my own reputation, not to mention this book in your hands.

The reason is simple. The impetus behind this book, its focus from the start, has been to list the benefits of puzzle-solving on the brain. And there's no point crowing cognitive gains, pledging how twisty clues can fire your neurons, if the science isn't there. The moment of truth has come. Today must be a success or this manuscript has been written in vain, my last 30 years of solving and setting puzzles a bum steer.

The crunch gets down to magnetism. Everywhere you look, from human-interest headlines to pop-psych pieces, there's talk of puzzles boosting your brain, how crosswords enhance lateral thinking, or why sudoku is a whetstone for logic—yet a key piece of evidence always seems missing. Where are the brain scans? The hard data? How do we know neurons sparkle until we see the images derived from an fMRI—a scanner responsible for functional magnetic resonance imaging? All those questions, quite separate from Renee's barrage, are the drivers behind this morning's trial, putting my brain on the line, and holding the central promise of this book to ransom.

'You're good to go,' says Renee. She puts down the clipboard and gestures to the door. I cinch my gown and follow her down a corridor, the lino cold on my feet. The passage forms part of the Florey Institute of Neuroscience and Mental Health, a winding path inside a grander maze, much like the brain itself, where the Austin Hospital in Heidelberg—in north-east Melbourne—encases one Florey lobe, that in turn enfolds the Brain Imaging Research Institute, where my tube of destiny awaits.

So, too, my neuro-trio. The tallest member is cognitive neurologist Associate Professor David Darby, a rangy man with salt-and-pepper stubble. His accomplices are Associate Professor David Abbott, another Florey brainiac, plus Dr Sarah Holper, who devised the protocol for today's pilot study.

'Are you ready?' asks David Darby.

'As near as I get.'

Next door, the tube resembles a sarcophagus. In a cryptic touch, my spirits lift to realise that 'Tesla'—part of the machine's name—is an anagram of my surname, speaking as the world's first hostage solver.

Renee sits me on the conveyor belt. It pokes like a shelf from the tube. She gives me earbuds to insert and next comes a hockey mask—*click, click*. The grille locks snugly across my face, like Hannibal Lecter's muzzle, all in the name of trailblazing.

'Here,' says Renee, producing a computer mouse, one to click in each hand. 'You know how this goes?' And I nod, recalling the protocol the neuro-team had devised in the weeks leading up to D-Day, where D stands for Discovery.

'Lie flat,' says Renee. The conveyor belt is cold along my spine. I feel a pillow prop my head, and then comes the horizontal mirror, a rear-view lozenge fixed across the bridge of my nose. Before I have a chance to renege, a secret button is jabbed, the belt rumbling my body deeper inside the tube.

Test clues come first, a dummy run to check if my mouse responses work—a left click to signal my recognition of the clue's formula, a right click to denote I've cracked it. Everything—the scanner and the mouse routine—seems to be in working order, my brain included. This paves the way for the clues that count, the experiment going 'live' as the timer starts pulsing, my heart starts racing, and the first official clue appears:

Organised relay in good time (5)*

The rest is a blur—yet not a blur. My senses drown in a stream of words and puns, a series of homophones and red herrings, every clue appearing on a screen behind my head, the letters written in reverse to suit my periscope fitting.

Don't worry if you're unfamiliar with the language of cryptic crosswords. This book will change that, as now there's every reason to read it. Yes, the risk paid off. Despite the alien setting and the creepy mask, my brain illuminated in combinations the researchers had never seen, for all their years of surveying images at the Florey. I'll let Sarah Holper explain:

'Nothing like this has been done before. Prior research has pinpointed what brain regions are active when you gaze at a loved one, or a tarantula. But that "aha" feeling when you solve a crossword clue: where does *that* come from, anatomically speaking? Is there a particular nub of brain responsible for that insight moment? That's what we wanted to find out. The real possibility was that we wouldn't find any special region. That the crossword-based "aha" moment was all in our heads, as it were.'

David Darby spells out the protocol: 'First we grilled David with 220 cryptic clues in rapid succession. Multiple images of his entire brain were taken every second of his 35-minute workout. Initially we were worried that we wouldn't have enough data, that David would be too slow to get through all the clues. Robust results required lots of "aha" moments to see if there was a common brain region active. We set a time limit of nine seconds per clue. If David solved it, he pressed on the right-hand mouse and the next clue appeared; if he timed out, the

---

* EARLY.

next clue appeared regardless. It was relentless. To our delight, David averaged 3.67 seconds to solve each cryptic clue.'

(Don't try this at home—or not yet. Not until you immerse your mind in *Rewording the Brain*, learning how to flex for a cryptic workout.)

Back to Dr Holper: 'At this point, after the cryptic workout, we had no idea if the experiment had actually worked. More data was needed. Hence the study's next phase, where we wheeled David back into the scanner for round two: 132 quick clues at the same tempo. These would act as controls, a means of spying on the brain when the challenge was pure semantics: *Young male horse* (4), *Mexican liquor* (7), and so on.'

COLT. TEQUILA. Back in the tube, my brain devoured the orthodox clues, clicking a single mouse as each answer leapt to mind. *Lone performer*—SOLOIST. *Picture in pieces*—JIGSAW. At their simplest, quick clues serve as reflex tests for habitual solvers, a vocab quiz requiring call and response.

Meantime, returning to the jigsaw of cryptic clues, three categories had been selected for the trial, as the Florey team explained once the scanning had been done. That first sample you met on the previous page used the anagram formula, while the other styles selected were homophone and pun. The variety was a way of analysing how my brain coped with different tricks, and a chance to compare the average times each formula took to unravel. For the record, my brain worked fastest with pun clues (3.14 seconds), followed by anagrams (3.85 seconds) and then homophones (3.98 seconds). These trends emerged in the subsequent data-crunching, as the Florey trio explained:

'After the trial, we had hundreds of thousands of images of David's brain in action. fMRI relies on tracking blood flow in response to changes in thinking. If you lift a dumbbell, blood gets diverted to your biceps to supply extra oxygen and glucose. The same is true when you exercise your brain: when you're using a particular area of brain, blood is diverted towards it. We sifted out the scans taken precisely at David's "aha" moments, set the computer whirring, and held our breath.'

'Amazingly, it worked,' declared Dr Holper. 'We found a unique brain region that activated at the exact moment when David solved a cryptic clue. A patch of brain just above his left eyeball. (The orbital surface of the left frontal lobe, technically.) It was dormant during solving, and never showed a flicker when failing to crack a given clue. But then when success arrived, the patch illuminated, dimly when solving a quick clue, and like a flame when David solved a cryptic clue, the lobe igniting at the moment of insight. It was all we had hoped for.

'From previous research, we know this brain region is important for emotional regulation. We identified some other brain regions that were particularly active during cryptic solving: areas behind both of David's eyebrows (the frontal poles) and a more central patch (the medial frontal lobe surfaces). The most recent expansion, evolutionarily, of our primate brain, the frontal poles are involved in exploring alternative courses of action, and complex problem solving, while that central patch is needed for impulse control.'

Dr Holper, a keen cryptic solver away from the clinic, lent her own insights on seeing the results: 'When you grapple with a difficult puzzle, you'll know this pattern of frustration and delight, how you need to check your emotions, or fight the urge to whoop when finding the answer. Thanks to this data, we now know that sensation is real. It's measurable.'

The tesla tube converted a pipe dream into a reality—evidently a cryptic habit can trigger some remarkable pinwheels in your skull. While deeper research needs be done, recruiting other solvers of varying experience, the experiment was nothing short of promising, exhilarating. Early analysis affirmed the anecdotal sense of cryptic clues stimulating the neurons in unique and particular ways—and this book explores the reasons behind those internal fireworks.

No matter which scan the team consulted, here was a brain in ferocious play, an opalescent lump of grey matter making lightning-quick connections, bypassing impasse, leaping on answers, just as your brain will match the lightshow with time and insight. The chance is yours. Regardless of your solving level, from tyro to virtuoso, *Rewording the Brain* is the book to recharge your neurons and set them loose in new directions. Across nine chapters, plus a string of clue-by-clue tutorials, followed by a bank of puzzles to conquer, this is the book to help you crack the cryptic code, as well as grasp why such a challenge will do your brain a power of good.

| I | N | T | R | O | D | U | C | T | I | O | N |

Sir Arthur Conan Doyle, the creator of Sherlock Holmes, compared the human brain to an empty attic, with one catch: 'You have to stock it with such furniture as you choose.'

Neuroscientists may dispute the 'empty' side of things—a living brain might seem inert to the naked eye but it's never empty. No clinician worth their salt, however, would quibble that ours is the power to furnish the room upstairs, equipping the brain with fresh ways of thinking—the idea central to this book. Whether you load your cranium with detective novels or music, maps or Grand Prix races, the input will influence how you see the world, and how your brain operates.

Puzzles alone can shape your grey matter in surprising ways, as those Florey snapshots have only begun to suggest. A simple matchstick array, for instance, can sharpen your spatial smarts. A sudoku grid is tailor-made to hone your logic, pushing the bounds of what-if algebra well past the grid's confines. Anagrams can blend your powers of language dexterity and problem-solving as much as blending letters. And then there are the lateral leaps involved in a cryptic crossword, furnishing the attic with fittings you've never even imagined.

All these pursuits occupy Part One of *Rewording the Brain*, as we grapple with the why behind the puzzle impulse: why our brains are attracted to wordplay and other deceptions in the first place, and why the habit of solving conundrums has multiple benefits for Doyle's room upstairs.

Part One will also reveal how an appetite for puns can encourage an inventive mindset. We'll take time to road-test quick and cautious thinking, seeing how puzzles can boost both modes, and why they enhance daily resolutions. We'll also explore how cryptic language boosts the knack of connecting and disconnecting concepts both small and large: one more avenue towards a lither brain.

More than memory or focus or strategic savvy, puzzles can deliver subtle advantages. To understand these in real terms, we'll call on the latest studies from home and abroad, playing jazz and obsessing over blackberries, visiting an amnesiac called HM plus a lovable crossword class, unlocking research that maps the way we humans have flourished as insightful animals.

Flourished and endured—with census data indicating some 15 per cent of Australians are now over 65, a portion translating as close to four million people. Projections suggest that figure will reach 8.7 million by 2056. Yet growing older doesn't always mean growing better; brains age in tandem with their owners. The cortex—or outer layer—thins. Plasticity abates. Neural links can slow over time. And the older we get, the more we live with the spectre of dementia.

But we can make an active difference and lend our brains every chance to keep pace with an evolving world. How might puzzles—and other brain games—help us? Can a crossword a day really keep the fog at bay? Part One aims to illuminate what the latest findings tell us.

Over the next ten chapters we'll enter the brain itself, starting with a virtual tour. Or at least, we will as much as anybody can: even among experts, like British neuroscientist Susan Greenfield, the brain remains 'the final frontier in human understanding'. In a space the size of a match-head, say, the brain plays host to as many as a billion neural connections, teeming with activity. In a short while we'll learn the nature of this tumult and how we might enhance its powers via puzzling.

No sooner will you learn of the brain's floorplan and functions—the secrets behind deduction and intuition—than you'll reach a second mystery, better known as cryptic crosswords. Gobbledegook to some people, addictive delight to others, the cryptic clue in all its shapes and sizes will be unravelled in Part Two, the book's other hemisphere if you like, the How-To succeeding the Why. There I'll equip you with the art of clue-conquering, sharing the lowdown on the cryptic genre's formulas—from anagrams to charades, from homophones to reversals—telling you how to spot them and how to pounce.

That said, you may already be a seasoned solver. If so, feel free to leapfrog Part Two, although I'd advise otherwise, since tucked away in this segment is a celebration of the craft's finer points, outlining the rarer traps you may meet in the land of Cryptopia. Rookies and veterans alike will glean insights galore, and meet some spectacular clues as examples.

After the tutorial comes the party that embodies Part Three: a suite of 50 puzzles to extend your brand-new talents. Part Three—the cerebellum annexed to the book's two hemispheres—is an original crossword collection arranged from friendly to gnarly. First come the samplers, mini-grids devoted to certain cryptic recipes, and later a procession of mixed clues, with sneak-peek options to reveal each clue type in case the going gets too tough.

Beyond that, in the coda of puzzles to conclude the book, you'll be solving solo. Maybe you won't crest the highest peak this time around, but you'll definitely learn the reasons why the striving counts, as well as grow familiar with the ground rules. Regardless of the heights you climb, your grey matter will thank you, not just today, but every day you wrestle with a puzzle. *Rewording the Brain* is the book to explain why, as well as show you how.

PART ONE

THE
WH[Y]

How puzzling nourishes your neurons

LET THE BRAIN TOUR BEGIN

The brain is the body's command centre, the headquarters in our head. Scary when you consider how small it seems, weighing roughly 1.3 kilograms, compact enough to perch in a cupped palm. Yet the key word here is *compact*. While the organ may resemble a small parboiled cabbage, there is a lot to see if you know where to look.

Take the outer layer encasing the cabbage's bulk. This is the cortex, Latin for 'bark', the actual grey matter we use as colloquial shorthand for the brain itself. The cortex is responsible for all manner of vital functions, from memory to attention, from language to awareness: the core skills a puzzle demands. It's no thicker than leather, only 2.5 millimetres deep on average, but critically, unlike leather, the cortex is convoluted: a crinkled mass of ridges (gyri) and furrows (sulci), plus the deeper indents known as fissures. Together, these corrugations allow humans to out-think any other species. Courtesy of crinkling, we can even keep a few moves ahead of chimpanzees, whose brains, while superficially humanoid, contain fewer convolutions, meaning three-quarters less surface area should the cabbage ever be pulled taut.

Size, of course, isn't everything. This is especially true for intelligence, when trying to gauge a creature's smarts by virtue of their brain's weight and mass. A sperm whale's brain, say, is six times heavier than ours. This is impressive, sure, but the more meaningful metric is the body-to-brain-mass ratio, and here Moby Dick fares poorly. Dolphins and humans, on the other hand, have much denser cortices.

Furthermore, this density is twofold, the cortex encased by a left and a right hemisphere. To the naked eye the hemispheres seem identical, and yet each of us has a degree of lateral dominance, a workload bias across the divide. Nine in ten right-handers, for example, have their speech centres located in the left hemisphere, and the remaining one in ten in the right. By contrast, 65 per cent of left-handers have speech centres in the left, a further 20 per cent are located in the right, and the remainder claim bilateral speech centres. That's just a single snapshot of our inner complexity, and each brain is unique, with its own maze of pathways and hubs. But for now, let's continue with our tour.

The cortex is sealed together by a fibrous band called the *corpus callosum*, or 'tough body'. Just as sticky-tape adheres to giftwrap, this C-shaped strip runs from nose to nape, both fastener and neural thoroughfare between the hemispheres.

Digging deeper, we enter the inmost lobes, the four segments making up the cerebrum, the brain's upper bulk, where each precinct has its own set of roles to play.

If one lobe is the boss, then the frontal lobe is your forerunner. Occupying the skull's anterior arc, that curve above your brow, this segment governs many of the body's voluntary movements. This includes walking and also where to walk, as the prefrontal cortex is tied up with decision-making as well as problem-solving. Mood and speech are also traced here, making this segment a cornerstone of who we are.

When comparing the evolution of species over millennia, humans have enjoyed the greatest expansion in this brain segment. Since antiquity, the feline brain's frontal lobe has only expanded by 3 per cent, against a massive 29 per cent in our own species. *Homo sapiens*, it could be said, climbed to the top of the zoological pile thanks to that development.

Below the prefrontal cortex is the temporal lobe, named for the skull's two temples that defend the area. Language dwells here, in tandem with the senses, notably hearing. New memories are captured here too. Time and deeper processing may etch these so-called working memories into established data, whether that's declarative (recalling a name, a fact) or procedural (like riding a bike). More on both later, in the chapter 'Memory'—for now, let's keep the tour rolling.

Climbing back into the upper reaches, at the rear of the skull you'll find the parietal lobe. The word stems from *'paries'* in Latin, or 'wall'. As you're reading this sentence, the parietal is in full swing, as focus mainly dwells here. Numbers and logic swim nearby too, along with language, a crossover from the temporal, in league with sorting sensory input from touch to taste. Pain is registered here as well. And when gurus advocate mindfulness—see the chapter 'Focus'—the parietal is the one lobe we most heavily draw upon.

Last lobe but not least is the occipital. Despite sitting furthest from your eyes, lining the posterior bulge above your nape, this brain section supervises sight. The same lobe also handles spatial duties, the kind you'll need for the upcoming matchstick puzzles. In keeping with space and sight, the occipital—Latin for 'the back of the head'—is also vital in recognising shapes and colours, making this bundle of neurons the skull's fashionista of the foursome.

However, neat as any cranial diagram strives to be, the brain can adjust and reinvent itself. This is the concept of neuroplasticity, theorised in the last fifty years. Should damage occur to one lobe, another lobe might well compensate over time, forging new circuitry to bypass the deficit. Likewise, to say that memory, for one, resides in a single lobe is to ignore the constellation effect at large in the brain, where recall is steeped throughout the network. Aside from the survival basics located in the hindbrain alone—the reptilian pith in charge of breathing and heartrate, wakefulness and sleep—there is no fixity within the infinity.

So there you have it, the basic itinerary. I've neglected several key regions—notably the hippocampus and so-called subcortical level, including the basal ganglia and thalamus (the system's sensory router, which we'll meet at various points in the chapters to come). Nevertheless, I hope you have a better understanding of your attic's layout now—a grey-blueprint of your brain—before we explore the same organ under pressure, seeing how your cabbage copes (and flourishes) with the input of puzzles.

Neural pathways

Q: What's the difference between brain and mind?

Not a riddle, but a genuine question. Often we use the two words interchangeably, but they are in fact distinct: the brain is the physical organ, while the mind is its mental dimension, what we *do* with our skull's contents. American novelist Jeffrey Eugenides believes, 'Biology gives you a brain. Life turns it into a mind.'

Or, if you like, the brain is the hardware to the mind's software. Memory, insight and every other function comprise the programs, so to speak—specific tasks performed by the cerebrum. In the meantime, the components—the folds and fissures and *corpus callosum*—entail the organic hardware. You can't have one without the other. Both are there to serve its ally, which is why the words are often swapped, except in the anatomy lab.

The reason I make this distinction is to help you think about thinking, the mechanics behind cognition. We peered deep inside our skulls a moment ago to reveal the city map inside our heads. But what about the traffic? How does a burnt finger send pain to the parietal lobe? How does a riddle, once heard, arrive in the temporal region, level with your eyebrow, then pass upwards to the problem-solving frontal lobe?

A vital component is axons, wisps of fibre running the length of cells, serving as chutes for the incoming signals. But the heroes are the neurons. You have some 100 billion of them in your cortex, and each carry their own relay equipment. To receive signals, every neuron owns a set of tiny branches radiating from either end, called the dendrites. Named after tree in Greek, the dendrites serve as receivers, awaiting any trace of the brain's electrical flow.

In simple terms, this electricity is generated by a constant imbalance of ions. At rest, neurons have negatively charged innards. An incoming signal sparks the opening and closing of ion-channel floodgates, transiently flipping the internal charge to positive. This change in voltage is called the action potential, faithfully relaying the message.

Amazing, don't you think? All these invisible transactions go on to not only solve a jigsaw, *per se*, but en masse they could also power a low-watt bulb. To further your amazement, every neuron is isolated by the tiniest gap, some 20 nanometres wide—a gap we call the synapse, making the neurons one vast archipelago.

Synapse, I should explain, derives from '*synapsis*' in Greek, or 'connection'. But how can a gap translate as a connection? How can neurons communicate if each cell is marooned by its own private moat?

The answer lies in neurotransmitters. An action-potential surge streaks from a neuron cell body to the outermost tips of its axon, stirring the neurotransmitters into life. Much like chemical couriers, the transmitters loiter at the end of the axons, working as messengers-for-hire across the extracellular fluid.

As the neuron emits electricity, the transmitters kick into action, including amino acids and peptides, or what I call the mule molecules. (Hmm, the mulecules?) As a thought flashes across the cerebrum, these proteins are recruited, and different chemicals react to different charges.

Multiply that action a million times, a billion times, and you have a picture of your brain at work. And at play. Let's say I asked you to name Santa's nine reindeers. Countless neurons would spark into action, the entire pathway a warp-speed alternation of neural signals, switching from electrical to chemical in nature, all in the name of retrieving trivia. I only hope you get the answer right.

The more we learn about the brain—the least trivial thing we own—the more questions we generate. In the grand scheme of things, neuroscience is a relative newcomer compared to other disciplines. In the Iron Age, around 500BC, humans believed the brain did nothing more than cool the blood. Now we know the brain to be a universe we're only just beginning to map, an evolutionary marvel that guards its secrets closely. Study by study, however, we are gaining more clues, deciphering the wonder, learning how to use it more wisely. To renew it. To maximise it. And in that spirit lie the challenges at the core of each coming chapter, where we turn to puzzles to understand the inmost puzzle that is the brain.

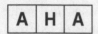

The euphoria of eureka

Stephen Sondheim adores cryptic clues—or British-style clues, as they're called in his neck of the woods. The American composer puts it this way: 'The nice thing about doing a crossword puzzle is you know there is a solution.'

Eventually, presuming you persevere. Because some solutions don't come fast; you need to stalk them, shake them into sight, presuming an answer comes at all.

Or you surrender. I mean, why not? Waving the white flag requires a lot less strain than torturing the neurons for an hour. If the puzzle is part of a book, flick to the back to check the answer. If the puzzle appears in the newspaper, wait until tomorrow to fill in those blank squares.

Yet stubborn solvers don't, and one big reason why is called the 'aha' rush. You know the answer exists, so you persist. You scratch a little deeper until you relieve the itch.

Take a so-called quick clue from Joon Pahk, a freelance compiler for the *New York Times*, the city that's home to Sondheim. Pahk's puzzle ran a few years back, including this innocuous clue:

Number of holidays?

The answer has five letters. At the time, trying to fill the grid, I suspected THREE was the answer. Or SEVEN. How many holidays in a calendar year? EIGHT?

Or maybe the clue had a sardonic edge, prompting the likes of ZILCH or I WISH. (Puzzles in America don't give an answer's letter count, aside from the number of squares allocated within the grid. Nor do US clues indicate if the answer is a phrase, entailing several words.

Hence I WISH or IN TOW might occupy five blanks.) Then again, perhaps QUOTA was the so-called holiday number, one's allotted rest-days in the working year. Even LEAVE seemed plausible, the number of holidays you accrue. By this stage you're right to suspect the clue was innocuous only on the surface.

As much cryptic as quick, Pahk's wording aims to sidetrack your brain, sending it down the wrong path. Either you surrender and check the answer, seeing where you were fooled, or you hold your nerve, knowing the blissful aha rush will reward your effort.

Cryptic crossword solving comes down to faith on two levels. First your faith in the setter, believing their solution will be worth the trouble of seeking. And second, the faith in your own neurons, trusting that the answer can be summoned from your neural HQ. To fuel this twofold faith is the prospect of a 'eureka' moment. Even if you've never solved a crossword, a kenken or a logic puzzle, I guarantee you've already experienced the glee a breakthrough brings. You face a problem; you reach an impasse; the answer seems unreachable, until you rethink the situation and *bang*—the high arrives. Not only does a problem get fixed or a puzzle completed, but your brain feels fulfilled.

But why? What triggers the brain's sudden insight, and why does the brain seem so charged when that eureka finally arrives?

It's time then to examine this aha moment—that occupational pleasure among solvers—as well as the genesis of insights in general. Facing a dilemma or a difficult clue, how does our brain turn a brick wall into a light bulb?

And if you're still not sure about Joon Pahk's clue, don't fret. The answer will arrive before this chapter's end, whether by my hand, or by your grey matter. But first, to understand aha, we need to play with matches.

Houston, we have a problem

One day in Texas, Bhavin Sheth was playing with matches. Less in a pyro way than a neuro way. The plan was to use the props as a means of measuring brainwaves.

Dr Sheth, an associate professor in neuroscience at the University of Houston, was using a series of puzzles to monitor how solvers solve, to chart how neurons work under pressure, and trace the buzz of that glorious aha.

His guinea pigs were students selected from campus. The puzzles were a series of cognitive tests, from lateral to lexical, from easy to unorthodox, just like the matchstick puzzle below. On the table, the equation didn't make sense:

$$XI + I = X$$

Translated from the Roman numerals, the sequence reads:

$$11 + 1 = 10$$

Which it doesn't. Even a toddler could tell you that. Opening the way to Dr Sheth's question: how do you correct the sum, moving as few sticks as possible, and still keep 10 as the solution?

The crunch is *moving as few sticks as possible*. The obvious remedy would be to simply move the second match, transforming the equation in one tweak to:

$$IX + I = X$$

It's neat, but Sheth encouraged the students to look harder. Smarter. There was a simpler way, he promised. To measure how the solvers coped, Sheth harnessed each student to an electroencephalogram, or EEG. Imagine a hairnet made of cables, where each cable links to a pair of electrodes placed on the scalp. As a pair, the electrodes will vary by what voltage they receive via the brain, this fluctuation charted in peaks and troughs on the screen. Professor Sheth studied these waves as his students wangled matches.

And wangled. And wangled. They tried a dozen approaches— altering symbols, turning Xs into Vs, editing the maths symbols—but none could imagine how anything could be more minimal than the single move shown above.

This narrowness of thinking is a symptom of functional fixedness, as the mindset is known. Too often we observe things in a prescribed light, as if one scenario demands one outlook, and one outlook only. Such thinking forfeits the potential of multiple perspectives, stuck in one groove at the expense of smarter ways.

For example, if I write the word FLOWER, what do you think of? Possibly blooms spring to mind—or spring itself. You might picture daisies and tulips, wreaths and bouquets, kindergarten drawings or an ikebana bowl. Yet how many people entertain the idea of something that flows, literally a FLOW-ER?

That is fixedness at work. We cling to unique interpretations despite others existing. We prefigure an answer and make every effort to reach it, striving to match our perceptual bias regardless of other potential answers. In the same way, we'll gaze at 9, the figure, seldom conceiving how the same squiggle can represent 6 with a twist of the wrist. Thanks to fixedness, we think too heavily along one tangent, deepening a rut out of routine. Concentration like this can be both blessing and curse. Solvers need to focus to fix a problem, yet not fixate to the point of lethargy. Sri Lankans know the syndrome as *kupa-manduka*, or frog in the well, where a stricture of thinking equates to a narrowness of perspective, just as the frog in the well can only observe a tiny circle of sky rather than the sky's true width.

The idiom holds true in problem-solving. Stare too hard at any conundrum and you're likely to be blinded by a single viewpoint. Even the word concentration implies a clustering, the word implying a pooling of perspective, a centralised bunching of resources, as if every conscious thought is jammed through one funnel.

Back in Houston, Bhavin Sheth observed the students' brainwaves were dominated by gamma waves, the common 'tell' of concentration. The gamma pattern calls the brain to attention, sweeping the lobes front to back some forty times per second, the rhythm depicted on the EEG's screen.

For all the focus, however, the students were getting nowhere. Did they read the instructions correctly? Quote, unquote: can you correct the sum, moving as few sticks as possible, and still keep 10 as the solution?

$$X| + | = X$$

I've already given you several hints about the answer, but if you need a little more encouragement, I vote we switch from matches to music.

Jazz detour

Dr Charles Limb, jazz musician and surgeon, is based at the University of California. He likens our brain to the cosmos, an inner space no less bewildering than the galaxies beyond us. One key tool to help us grasp this neural universe, the field's own telescope in a sense, is the fMRI tube, a device I've come to know personally.

Several steps advanced from an EEG, functional Magnetic Resonance Imaging relies on blood flow, as the Florey experiment illustrated. An active bit of brain needs more oxygen, delivered by blood, than a less active brain portion. In essence, the fMRI detects these distinctions, charting where oxygen is in peak demand, and which parts of the brain are relatively idle. While the fMRI still has drawbacks—its din, the terror its confines hold for claustrophobics—Limb deems the tube the best tool in the shop, a prized means of mapping our brains' points of light, just as ancients had charted the constellations.

Rather than puzzle-solving, Limb's focus was on improvisation, inviting jazz musicians to carry a tune into score-free territory. 'Artistic creativity—it's magical, but it's not magic,' as Limb put it. 'Meaning that it's a product of the brain.' As both scientist and muso himself, Limb was intrigued to see the mental genesis of creative solutions.

He was relying on BOLD imaging, just as Associate Professor David Darby and his team had opted to use for the cryptic trial. BOLD stands for blood-oxygen-level-dependent imaging. Whenever a neuron needs energy, it draws oxygen and sugar from the blood. This transaction is captured by the fMRI, allowing scientists to see which lobes are doing the greater toil, almost like a traffic update for a metropolis.

Which precinct then would host the heaviest 'jam' when it came to musical jamming? That was the question to test as Mike Pope, a jazz

MATCH SETS

Will your neurons be nimble enough to solve these six spatial puzzles? The answers appear on page 15.

Puzzle 1
Remove three matchsticks to
make the equation true.

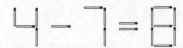

Puzzle 2
Here are six matches. Add five
more and make nine.

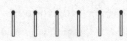

Puzzle 3
Move three matchsticks to make
three equilateral triangles.

Puzzle 4
Can you move three matches so
that there are four triangles?

Puzzle 5
Move four matchsticks to make
three squares.

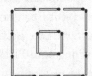

Puzzle 6
Here are two wine glasses, built
from ten matchsticks. Can you
move six of these to build the
house that holds the glasses?

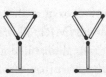

guru with a zeal for improvisation, squeezed inside an fMRI tube in Dr Limb's clinic. Tightening the squeeze was a toy-sized keyboard laid across Pope's thighs, a baby piano with special powers: instead of producing notes, the keyboard absorbed finger pressure. Pope was asked to respond to some jazz, a series of exploratory riffs from Limb himself on an orthodox keyboard outside the scanner.

Picture the scene, a jazz club in a clinic, musicians in lab coats. Limb played four bars as a stimulus for Pope's response, the subject fluidly pressing his keys inside the tube, replying with silent music. To sustain the interplay, Pope's music was instantaneously translated into audible phrasings via software so that Dr Limb could respond, and so on. The two men traded music with abandon, winding between minor and major keys, generating ahas aplenty as the melody wandered. But instead of sharing a stage, half of the duo lay prone in a magnetic field, his every neural flare-path logged for posterity.

The initial data sketched an astonishing picture. Two things in particular caught Limb's eye. The first was the intense activity in 'Broca's area', a pocket in the frontal lobe named after Paul Broca, a French physician who plumbed the mysteries of speech production 150 years ago. This indicated music is a grammar as much as any other tongue, a semantic system of octaves and semiquavers.

The second revelation related to darkness. Our metaphors for aha moments are insistently suffused with light—a bulb ignites above our head, scales fall from our eyes, allowing us to see the light, the truth. Yet Mike Pope's brain-map told a different truth. Throughout the riffing, the subject's medial prefrontal cortex was ablaze. This brain segment, level with the hairline, is linked to decision-making: a driver reflexively choosing a freeway lane without conscious thought, the solver's impulse to move a match. But as jazz filled the clinic, Pope's lateral prefrontal cortex was largely idle, a car sitting in neutral. This region is central to introspection. If the BOLD screens were any guide, Pope was hardly aware of being Pope as he played. His self-reflection was all but asleep, the blankness all the more dramatic when compared to the fireworks in the adjacent region, the medial prefrontal cortex vested with self-expression.

MATCH SETS

Did you manage to match wits?

Puzzle 1
Thanks to Matchstick Puzzles at
<http://matchstickpuzzles.
blogspot.com.au>

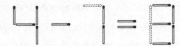

Puzzle 2
Maxey Brooke, *Trick, Games
and Puzzles with Matches* at
<www.arvindguptatoys.com/
arvindgupta/matchplay.pdf>

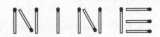

Puzzle 3

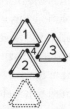

Puzzle 4
Designed by the Grabarchuk family,
<http://grabarchukpuzzles.com> via
<http://matchstickpuzzles.
blogspot.com.au/>.

Puzzle 5
Puzzle supplied by Mike Daigneault
via <www.learning-tree.org.uk/
stickpuzzles/stick_puzzles_old.htm>.

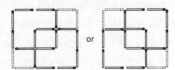

Puzzle 6
Courtesy of <www.puzzles.com/
PuzzlePlayground/TheWineGlasses/
TheWineGlasses.htm>.

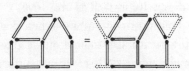

Hard conclusions are yet to be drawn from Limb's work, but the inference is clear. In order to create new solutions, some neurons need muzzling as much as others need unleashing—introversion must give way to the daredevil who doesn't blush at making mistakes. Find the off switch in one brain zone and you empower the other.

But how do you do that? If you wish to arrange notes, or grapple with crossword clues, how can you get your neurons to cooperate? Let's go back to that problem in Houston, with what we know now.

Perfect matches

Any luck with those matches? Or the so-called number of holidays? Keep the jazz musicians in mind, the way Mike Pope's brain suppressed its executive control to access a wilder sense of play. If the muso made a blunder, pressed the wrong key, the melody swept along regardless. There was no harm in thinking loose.

Back in Houston, Bhavin Sheth noted the more that gamma waves ruled their brains, the further the students stalled—their matches intact, the elegant solution unseen. $XI + I = X$ seemed etched in stone. We know some tried to move a match, making $IX + I = X$, which was admirable, but even that tweak could be surpassed. Yet how?

My first hint came a short while back, talking about 9 becoming 6 if you adopted a novel viewpoint. The second hint was the jazz experiment, seeing two musicians quit the score and treat music as an open space to move within. The technical term is restructuring, where your brain relents its fixity. In a sense, you sublimate the problem, placing the focal point offstage, out of sight, yet keeping the puzzle's challenge active in your working memory. You look elsewhere, in a way. Think otherwise. Because to experience that elusive aha, you need to be digressive as well as obsessive.

You must concentrate—then deviate. I'm sure you've noticed how many great ideas emerge out of daydreams, a dog walk, a prolonged shower, when daily cares are suppressed, even as your subconscious quietly toils on. The archetype of this is Archimedes, the genius lying back in his bath. The moment the water rose as he sank, the Greek happened upon the law of displacement, a problem he'd been gnawing at for ages. His resting brain solved what his fixated brain could not.

The students of Houston were nearing the same moment. Staring at matches can only get you so far. Besides, the matches were not the ones in need of changing. The equation could stay intact on the table. Only the observers were obliged to refresh their perspective.

Eureka. A few seconds before each solver solved the matchstick puzzle, a calmer theta wave pattern washed over the screen and the gamma waves dissipated. Compared to the busy gamma undulations, theta is more a level sea—the calm tidal tempo often bearing the insight that's been elusive for so long.

Along with the shift in wave patterns, Sheth observed a spot fire deep in the brain on the EEG monitor. This neural activity centred on the limbic cortex, the centre of emotional regulation lying astride the thalamus.

But that wasn't all. Thanks to BOLD imaging, Sheth could see a disco-like flashing in the *anterior cingulate* area of the limbic cortex, a band that fringes the *corpus callosum*. The *anterior cingulate* is deemed an important zone for impulse control, as well as the precinct that anticipates reward. In effect, the brain was changing its framework, relinquishing focus for freestyle thinking.

Houston, we have a solution. The answer to the matchstick problem relied on inverting the equation, or *changing sides at the bench.*

This was the rethink: finding a visuospatial solution to a mathematical problem. Realigned, the new sum asserted $X = I + IX$, which was true, the total unchanged, and not one match in need of moving.

$$X = I + IX$$

Which leaves us with one more puzzle to solve, namely Joon Pahk's clue: *number of holidays?* Any theories? These stories of improvised music and inverted matches should urge you to read the words in a different light. Number can mean several things apart from 1, 2, 3.

Just as flowers can flow, numbers can numb. That was my eventual response when solving Pahk's puzzle, entering the all-numbing BOOZE into the squares. Alcohol is a popular source of anaesthesia after all. But why did Pahk specify the holidays? That element didn't quite gel, goading my brain to stray in a new direction even as I ventured deeper into the crossword. When a C arrived as the answer's initial, I toyed with COUNT. Or maybe CROWD—streets are often swamped by extra numbers during the holidays. But then I saw the light—or the darkness set in.

I imagine that gamma waves stilled in tandem with the dimming of self-awareness, a muting of that insistence upon one interpretation . . . I read the clue as if for the first time. My mind switched over. The narrow-sighted frog fled the well. Suddenly 'Jingle Bells' rang a different bell, as I realised holidays referred to a particular holiday, and *number* was neither integer nor intoxicant, but something closer to a jazz tune. *Number of holidays*—the Christmas holidays, to be exact—is a CAROL.

These puzzles—a spatial trick and a sly piece of wording—channelled so many brains in so many false directions. In the end the answers lay in the art of fresh thinking, turning the tables, widening the frame. Yet that's just part of the cognition story. To learn a little more, to see the aha itself from a new perspective, let's look at tempo, and see how puzzles help the brain shift gears.

T E M P O

Pouncing versus pacing

The word tempo may feel out of place in a book devoted to the brain—and perhaps more in tune with melody masters like Mike Pope and Stephen Sondheim—but don't be too fast to judge. That's the gist in fact: thinking fast and thinking slow. Presto and lento. Your brain can do both well, but results may vary since there's a time for speed and a time for caution. To illustrate the point, take a closer look at the puzzle below. See if the trios loosen any thoughts:

1. BUMP   EGG   STEP
2. PINE   SAUCE   CRAB
3. BULLET   TOILET   ROAD
4. WALL   BACK   CLIP

Each threesome is united by a fourth word you need to determine.

Professor Mark Beeman, now chair of psychology at Illinois' Weinberg College at Northwestern, devised the puzzle back in 2004, asking volunteers to name the missing word per set, a word that could complete a compound word or phrase with all three members.

GOOSE is your first answer, for instance, making goosebump, goose-egg and goosestep. In trio number two, APPLE comes to the rescue, making pineapple, apple sauce and crabapple.

Notice the departure? Every goose-phrase carries the missing word in the first position, while in the apple trio the absentee is first *or* last. Your brain should now be on high alert. Extra wary, you'd be wise to reread those instructions: what missing word per set can make a compound word or phrase with all three members?

Now the ambiguity is evident: for each line, the missing word makes a compound, whether the keyword sits to the left or the right. Chances are your quick-thinking self neglected that detail, or made a false presumption. A rapid response can attract those problems, skimming the instructions, ignoring the manual, second-guessing what is needed. But then again, a rapid response can often solve a puzzle too. Could that be the case with trio number three—BULLET, TOILET and ROAD?

Either you saw the answer in a flash or you're still in the dark. Intuition is a mercurial force. You and I know the power as gut instinct, while scientists such as psychologist Daniel Kahneman prefer the term of System-1 thinking—a quick and often subconscious way of operating. A Nobel laureate in economics, Kahneman coined the term some ten years ago to distinguish between two modes of cognition: the instantaneous System 1 and the more deliberate System 2. Both systems come with their own rewards.

(Have you nabbed Beeman's BULLET trio yet?)

Operating a few degrees past word puzzles, Albert Einstein was trying to grasp the interconnection between time and space. The conundrum prompted him to say, 'There is no logical way to the discovery of these elemental laws. There is only the way of intuition, which is helped by a feeling for the order lying behind the appearance.' A feeling? That's what he said, one of history's greatest scientists, talking about that sneaky sensation we register even when a problem seemingly calls only for logic.

So what is this feeling? How does System-1 thinking play out in the brain? And why do intuitive decisions metaphorically reside in the gut, of all places? Surely the brain is the seat of insight, not your duodenum.

Sorry, I've been priming you, choosing words like gut and seat to make you ponder TOILET almost unthinkingly. The missing word is TRAIN, as in *bullet train, toilet train* and *road train*. And again, this third trio takes the puzzle one step further from the apparently simple instructions: not only can the missing word sit flush left or right (okay, we can ditch the toilet allusions now), but it can also be different parts of speech. TRAIN is a noun in two of the compounds, and a verb in the other.

This added complexity makes reaching the answers even harder, if you wish to approach Beeman's puzzle logically. Logic and reason, the natural enemies of intuition, are System-2 thinking, the stuff of analysis and protocol, a more conscious and deliberate mode. And more Neolithic too, beyond the animal impulses of System 1.

(Have you matched the final three by the way? WALL, BACK and CLIP? I'll leave the clock running and tell you in a page or two.)

With gamma waves flowing, the System-2 thinker would meticulously work through each trio and recite all the variants in working memory: silver bullet, magic bullet, bullet point, rubber bullet, and so on, until an eligible candidate emerges. Nor is there anything wrong with that left-brain approach—that's where such thinking mainly dwells. Much like an auditor, the System-2 thinker confirms every fact.

Comparatively, System 1 is a prehistoric flash, reaching a decision before it has time to be articulated. Gut feelings, to use the misnomer, largely ignite the right side of the brain, plus the limbic band deep within the cerebrum, our older core and home of emotions and long-term memory. You'll remember this patch from Sheth's experiment, the same segment flaring as students pounced on the matchstick puzzle solution.

Pounce. Flash. Wham. Strike. The verbs aligned with intuition all evoke speed. And speed, harking back to cave days, has been vital for survival. Our ancestors relied on their neural firing to sidestep crisis, or recognise danger as well as opportunity. And, more recently, to crack puzzles too.

After his word-trio puzzle, Professor Mark Beeman reached a conclusion that defied common sense: looking at each volunteer's hit-rate, in tandem with their solution time, and the readouts garnered from both EEG and fMRI devices, Beeman grew to see the quicker the answer came the more likely it was to be correct. Speed in this case was a solver's ally, as if the answer was being harpooned from the deep, rather than emerging through meticulous elimination. Beeman's study seemed to be clear: the faster the draw, the better your score.

But wait, aren't we taught to take our time when answering a question? Caution is every teacher's byword. And indeed, we should be cautious about this call to abandon caution. Let's take a closer look at tempo. If our brain is an engine, then we have two gears on offer, and both deserve to be engaged.

Fast and slow

Upon closer assessment of the puzzle data, Beeman discovered a clear divide emerged among the solvers. No matter the puzzle, the volunteers showed a bias towards one mode of thought over the other, System 1 versus System 2. The intuitive System-1 solvers displayed a flat pattern of neural activity, their cognition emerging from the right hemisphere and spreading across the neocortex like a swarm. Meanwhile, the analysts in the experiment—the System-2 thinkers—produced a cluster pattern limited to one region of the frontal lobe. By way of success, the intuitive camp enjoyed a 94 per cent hit-rate, while the System-2 crew only managed to achieve 78 per cent. Curious to add, 34 per cent of answers submitted at the last moment were wrong, in contrast to only 10 per cent of answers speedily given being incorrect.

Trust your gut seems the moral of the story, but not every scientist is taken by the precept. Enter Daniel Kahneman. In his milestone book *Thinking, Fast and Slow*, Kahneman argues that System-1 thinking is mainly reserved for minutiae, the everyday dilemmas of mustard or mayonnaise, window or aisle, blue socks or brown. Being so fast, and so efficient, intuitive thinking can seem autonomous, the inner voice that calls the shots.

System-2 thinking, however, is what we apply to the Big Decisions—matters of life and mortgages. As tempting as shortcuts seem, we tend to take the slower road to reach the bigger destinations. In a way, System 2 is our brain's handbrake, ensuring hunches don't lead to strife. Few of us buy a home on impulse. We don't swap careers on a whim. Instead we rationalise. We weigh the pros and cons. We overthink. In short, we filter the instincts embedded in System 1.

This is all well and good when choosing a college, a spouse, an insurance policy, but far less critical when it comes to seizing goose eggs. With little to lose you trust your gut, it seems. Though a brilliant experiment at Princeton in 2007 aimed to challenge that maxim: psychologists Adam Alter and Daniel Oppenheimer sought to test how our thinking changes as soon as stimuli are suppressed.

In their experiment, 40 students were handed a set of questions, including this teaser:

> A bat and a ball cost $1.10 in total.
> The bat costs $1.00 more than the ball.
> How much does the ball cost?

It's clear to read and just as simple to solve. So, what's your answer?

If you guessed 10 cents, then congratulations, you fell for the trap. Sound as that System-1 response might have seemed, your impulse was off-beam. Before you revise your answer, I want you to reread the puzzle, but now presented like so:

> A bat and a ball cost $1.10 in total.
> The bat costs $1.00 more than the ball.
> How much does the ball cost?

Harder to read, right? The reduction in point size was not a test of eyesight but a means of retarding a solver's perceptual fluency, the tempo it takes to perceive and understand a problem.

Across a series of puzzles, Alter and Oppenheimer discovered that nine in ten students bungled one such teaser when presented in a standard point size, yet the success rate soared the moment the point size shrank, or the text grew so faint it was barely legible.

Forced to decelerate, students got smarter. Errors dropped by a third. In short, when the brain was obliged to take the long road, its intuition was checked. System-1 thinking (reading the puzzle at speed) presumed the baseball cost 10 cents. But apply the brakes, thanks to the trouble in absorbing the question, and System-2 rightly reasoned the ball cost 5 cents.

So where does that leave us? When solving a puzzle, should we think fast or think cautiously? Will more success await the tortoise or the hare? The answer lies in the puzzle itself, as much as your own cognitive forte. Wise thinkers are aware of both approaches, as much as recognising the tempo that's historically yielded their better results, since there's no set speed when it comes to tackling problems.

Wallpaper, paperback and *paperclip* comprise the final set for Beeman's puzzle, whether that took you a second or a minute to reach. However, all this pales next to the complex puzzle of living, to facing the grander problems that life throws your way. Nonetheless, it pays to heed both modes—the fast and the slow, the intuitive and methodical. An agile brain is vital, capable of the swoop and the stab, but also has the ability to sift and verify.

Practice helps no end—the so-called 10,000 hours of singular devotion (to violins, to juggling, to crossword clues) that becomes a practitioner's second nature. Or to quote Einstein again, 'Creativity is the residue of time wasted.' After so many puzzles, whatever the puzzle, you recognise the traps. Over time, your brain develops its own gear ratio—the fast and the slow: when to follow your gut and when to be wary.

Puzzles in general help to calibrate those speeds. You will know yourself that every time you glimpse a Target puzzle, those jumble features in the paper, the nine-letter word will leap off the page in a blink, or take a good while of rearrangement. How will you fare with this one?

D E R
U H N
O G Y

Ten thousand hours of manipulating letters, or even a hundred hours, will deliver a fast-tracked answer via intuition. It must be HYDROGEN?

That's the peril of responding too soon. Not every pounce will find the prey. HYDROGEN is a miscount. There are times for speed and times to arrest your impulses. Going a little steadier, you incorporate the U and the upshot is GREYHOUND. In many ways the secret to solving—to thinking in general—is knowing which tempo to trust.

F O C U S

The endangered art of being present

Back in Houston we looked at concentration, the functional fixedness that can accompany acute focus. This time around, I put focus squarely into view, coming to the mindset's defence.

We'll also consider distraction—the antonym of focus—and how multitasking attracts its share of myths. And lastly, presuming your focus can hang in there, we'll also consider how mindfulness can arise from diversions, despite what diverting (the word) may suggest: that flawed notion of deflecting one's attention.

Historically, the word 'focus' hails from Latin where it meant 'fireplace', the heart as hearth if you like. In Caesar's day, focus was the home's central space, the source of warmth in Rome's long winters. Hub is a close cousin, this word deriving from Old English hob, or stove, the source of comfort drawing everyone closer.

It's ironic that the word focus is derived from a huddling of people, when the modern challenge of focusing lies more in isolating yourself from the intrusion of others. Because focus is perishable nowadays. Even as you read this paragraph, there's half a chance you're checking Facebook, or glancing to see if that email has arrived. If you're not, chances are you're still in a state of readiness, awaiting a ping. As I write this paragraph, my fingers are poised to switch from this document to my inbox, or to see which friend liked my holiday pic.

Welcome to the new millennium. Like it or not, our attention span is under siege.

Dr Bruce Morton, a researcher attached to Ontario's Brain and Mind Institute, measured the impact of shredded focus in 2015. Under lab conditions, Morton studied the brain activity of 112 subjects, in addition to surveying 2000 participants across Canada. The experiment's intent was to calculate the average length of the human attention span. Back in 2000, when similar research was conducted, the figure had been twelve seconds. Think about it—that's five shifts in focus every waking minute. But the bad news doesn't end there. Data from Morton's consequent experiment suggested that figure had lapsed to eight. We lost four seconds in fifteen years. By way of a yardstick, a goldfish is reputed to boast an attention span of nine seconds. It seems the attention span of the human animal—well, the human Canadian at least—is one second shy of your pet, Bubbles.

From the goldfish bowl to the office think-tank, the figures are no less telling. Back in the early 2000s, Professor Gloria Mark and her team from the Department of Informatics at the University of California observed workers at multiple finance and high-tech companies. Their goal was to tally the average number of distractions that occur across the workday.

Among the subjects were engineers, software developers, market analysts and project leaders, spread across a range of offices. Distractions could be anything from a spouse's SMS to a holiday pic to a colleague interrupting with project updates.

The magic figure they arrived at was three minutes—three minutes and five seconds to be precise: the interim between one interruption and the next. Of course, that interruption may have been self-triggered, a worker leaving her document mid-sentence to check her phone, or replenish her jasmine tea—any switch of focus that ushers her mind into a separate sphere.

And if the tally seems extravagant, then consider the impact of any distraction deemed as off-topic and exceeding two minutes. For example, if you're trying to complete an essay, and a family member intervenes with a logistic problem regarding carpooling, an issue demanding at least two minutes of your focus, then you may well need around 23 minutes and fifteen seconds to resume the initial task, as that can be the effect of a major jump off-topic, off-track. The burden is less about regathering your thoughts, and more to do with realigning your workload until focus and flow have had the chance to resume.

Furthermore, the informatics team learnt that a fifth of all disrupted jobs are left in limbo on any given day. You may have had every hope of completing report A by five o'clock, but that chore will now have to wait until tomorrow, thanks to the stream of intrusions.

This leads us to the modern myth of multitasking, that common boast among the super-parents and high-achieving execs. The evidence shows, however, that even when you're trying to do your best across several fronts, your brain struggles to succeed. Our slang recognises it, via such alternative labels as multislacking and multicrastinating. The ergonomic juggle of multitasking is, in fact, often only a matter of spreading your inefficiency across a range of focal points.

Multitask masters

Back in 2013, the *New York Times* commissioned two academics at Carnegie Mellon University to measure the actual brain drain that multitasking inflicts. Together, psychologist Eyal Peer and IT professor Alessandro Acquisti invited 136 volunteers to read a short passage, and then answer questions on the piece.

The volunteers were split into three groups. The first had nothing but the test to focus on, while the other groups were told they may well be contacted during the reading with further instructions.

And indeed, two interruptions waylaid groups two and three during the initial screening. But in a second appraisal—with identical group sizes, members and rules of engagement—there was one significant alteration: this time around, group three was *spared* the interruption, although still warned it might occur. The cohorts were labelled the Control Group, the Interrupted Group, and the Group on High Alert.

Given all those variants, which group would you expect to be more efficient? The results in many ways betray much about the state of modern life. In the first test, the two interrupted groups were 20 per cent 'dumber' than the control mob. That is, they botched an extra fifth of the questions, their focus the frailer for the interruptions as much as the distracted state that came with awaiting them.

The second time around, however, when group three was warned about an interruption but then spared the intrusion, their proficiency increased. Human beings seem to flourish when we recognise time

MIND TRAPS

Plenty of playground questions, shared by kids to trap unwary thinkers, happen to prey on our non-mindful ways. Take care when cracking these chestnuts, as the obvious answer won't be immediately obvious, owing to the way each conundrum is worded:

1. If a plane crashed on the border of France and Belgium, where would they bury the survivors?
2. David's dad has three sons: Snap, Crackle and who?
3. If there are five apples on a table, and you take away three, how many do you have?
4. Driving a bus, you count the people as they get on. At the first stop, four got on. At the second stop, two joined the bus, and one got off. And at the next stop, two got off. What colour are the driver's eyes?
5. Beware the sucker punch in this sequence's final question:
    (a) Acorns grow on what kind of tree? (Oak)
    (b) What stinky cloud comes from fire? (Smoke)
    (c) Harry Potter has an Invisibility . . . what? (Cloak)
    (d) What do you call the white part of an egg?

is fleeting, possible disruption a heartbeat away. Compare that to the swamp of doing ten things at once, where the brain will often battle to switch focus and fulfil any single task properly.

Research suggests our brains have grown to accept the daily onslaught of interruptions, toiling more feverishly in dread of the trill of an SMS, the knock at our cubicle, the Facebook Like. It's all at a cost, however. While our tempo might quicken, our stress levels spike too. And our intensity isn't guaranteed to produce anything more polished than our less harried colleagues who can often languish in the rarity of not being interrupted, wasting what surplus of time they enjoy as they anticipate the disruption that never occurs.

For all these reasons, academics tend to avoid using the term 'multitasking'. In a write-up of the Carnegie Mellon experiment, the preferred phrase was 'rapid toggling between tasks'. This might seem like splitting hairs, but the phrasing speaks more to the frenzy of the action, rather than as a pledge of its efficiency.

Does all this remind you of something? Aside from your daily chaos, I mean. Reading the results of these various experiments, I kept dwelling on one word. It's a sacred term of the early millennium, a catchword held dear for all the reasons thrown up by the research we've just been trawling. If focus was ever the basis of a new belief system, then that religion would be known as . . .

Mindfulness

Tess, my daughter, had to eat a blackberry in Year 12. Not the smartphone, the fruit. And when I say eat, I mean savour. Slowly. Teasing off each drupelet (those mini-sacs making up the berry) and rolling each parcel on the tongue. After a while, one by one, each drupelet would burst and she'd go back for another.

The exercise was overseen by a mindfulness consultant, a visitor to the school. His task was to train the school's senior students in flexing the 'attentional muscle', as he insisted on calling what we would otherwise call focus.

Known as the raisin exercise, this slo-mo consumption aims to muffle the brain's white noise, to channel the senses into a single task. As you ponder the fruit in your hand, in your mouth, your peripheral cares dwindle for a time.

Jon Kabat-Zinn is the creator of the Stress Reduction Clinic and the Center for Mindfulness, based in Massachusetts. He says, 'Mindfulness means paying attention in a particular way: on purpose, in the present moment, and non-judgementally.' Presence and tolerance are the two pillars of the practice. In tandem, they benefit our brain: a tolerant outlook helps to lower stress, while the exaggerated sense of presence boosts the endangered art of focus.

In a joint 2010 study, combining Sydney University and the Norwegian University of Science and Technology, researchers found a proliferation of alpha waves in the meditative mind. 'This wave type has been used as a universal sign of relaxation during meditation and

YOURS MINDFULLY

Numerous techniques can help you reach a mindful state. These include:

+ Monitor your breath – deep and rhythmic breathing is a useful practice to prepare for some of the techniques below.
+ Focus on a fixed object (the mandala principle) until your mind no longer wanders from the focal point. A candle is also useful: allow the image to imprint on your vision, and then close your eyes and hold the image.
+ Squeeze your hand, or pinch your forearm or leg, for twenty seconds. Then release your grip and concentrate on the body's subsiding memory of the action.
+ Immerse yourself in silence, even if that means earplugs.
+ Overhear your own thoughts, and see how readily you can minimise the 'I' in your subconscious drift, becoming a conduit rather than a protagonist.

Or why not convert your phone into an ally? There are many helpful mindfulness apps on the market, including Smiling Mind, Headspace, Buddhify, Calm, Simply Being and Stop, Breathe & Think.

other types of rest,' explained Norwegian Professor Øyvind Ellingsen. 'The amount of alpha waves increases when the brain relaxes from intentional, goal-oriented tasks. This is a sign of deep relaxation, but it does not mean that the mind is void.' Indeed, alpha waves denote a state of wakeful rest, a focused mode midway between sleep and fierce concentration.

Let us return to my daughter Tess. Her twenty-minute blackberry was simple compared to the next assignment: to ditch her phone for three days. To switch it off. Ignore it. Suddenly eating a blackberry felt like a picnic compared to boycotting an Apple. For the adolescents, the gadget ban went close to breaching Geneva conventions.

In fact, forget adolescents—I dare anyone under 65 to exist without their pocket lifeline. Business execs, busy parents, tradies, journalists . . . as a race we are iPhone clones, Samsung slaves, Nokia zombies.

The phone has come to represent our portable confidante, our oracle, our window on the world. The popular description of ditching your phone for a day, or living phoneless full stop, is a 'digital detox'—a favour for our brain.

Instead, take up a mindful habit—which one depends on you. Maybe yoga elicits a mindful state, or long-distance swimming. Perhaps it's finding time to stop and breathe deeply, lessening the body's natural steroid cortisol (the so-called stress hormone). Others turn to meditation, colouring books, the music of Bach, or dining on a single blackberry.

Or possibly your fix is a puzzle—your transfix, if you like—the mindfulness arising from absorption in a finite grid with infinite permutations. For many people, sudoku offers that pure focus, the clinical discipline of working with hypotheses. 'If this is 4, then that must be 3 or 8 . . .' But for me, that mandala is a crossword, a sentiment shared by Marcel Danesi, a professor of anthropology at the University of Toronto. Danesi describes the universal pull of puzzles as 'using your mind . . . to restore order from the chaos'. Perhaps I should leave that quote there, for Danesi adds: 'And once you have [restored order] you can sit back and say, "Hey, the rest of my life may be a disaster, but at least I have a solution."'

Puzzle-solving is focus plus reward. Regardless of the diversion, from code-breaking to anagram-making, a puzzle gathers every atom of your attention, with progress as affirmation and closure as reward. The fire of focus, in that Roman sense, can crackle at its most intense when dealing with a mental challenge that's actively designed to foil, an enigma reserving its solution only for those brains that can dwell on the task, to focus and potentially switch that focus in a new direction. Kenken or cryptic, a good puzzle is an invitation to freely associate ideas and theories, to speculate and troubleshoot, all within the call for fixity. Strange as it sounds, a solver can be lost and found at the same time—lost in the bafflement, and found in the sense of being thoroughly present, locked and alive in the conundrum. And in this era of shredded attention and meagre reward, that's powerful medicine.

M E M O R Y

Your brain as active archive

Wind back the clock to a minute ago. Now to a month ago. Now go back to your first day at school. It's clear that shimmering inside your cerebrum is a galaxy of dates and names. But how did we gain these details, and how do we retain them? And where do puzzles belong in this intricate mesh?

This chapter offers some tips on improving memory, from everyday shopping lists to Roman palaces. We'll also decode the electrochemical marvel that memory is, and meet a crossword addict called HM.

But first, see if you can memorise these twelve words:

cloud, thunder, breeze, emerald, ruby, diamond, mouth, foot, knuckle, goat, crab, lion

Strategic to a fault, your brain most likely bunched the words as you read them. Clustering or clumping is a proven technique, a way of sorting lengthy serves of data into logical bites. That's why credit card numbers are more easily remembered when broken into quartets. Compare that to memorising the hostile block of 0494227815296210. And no, you're not getting my three-digit security code.

To play along, now place your hand over the list of words above and see if you can recall any of the dozen. In order or at random, it doesn't matter.

How did you go? If you like, take a second look and try again.

Doubtless you fared better the second time around, thanks to the reinforcement of reading it twice, but also due to clustering: the twelve words were grouped into weather terms, gems, body parts and animals. (And not just any animals, but zodiac animals, each one four letters.) People with stronger memories will notice such quirks like these, making the words extra sticky.

RECOLLECTION RELICS

Culture depends on memory. This truth holds strong among ancient and indigenous cultures, especially those that flourished separate from any literary tradition.

Here in Australia, Aboriginal songlines preserve a narrative within the landscape, a chain of stories rooted to locations, just as Greeks built their cranial palaces where every turn and nook evoked a memory. Dot paintings and *tjuringa* (sacred totems of scored stone or wood) also act as memory maps, prompting primal knowledge to those who carry the traditions.

In central Africa, the *lukasa* fulfils a similar role. Deriving from the Luba people, the *lukasa* (or 'long claw') is sculpted from hardwood. Typically the object resembles a flattened hourglass, its surface adorned by nicks and embedded beads, a tactile autocue of stories readable to the select few.

Far less sticky is list number two, or what I call the Teflon Twelve:

glove, mattress, oyster, psalm, knight, squirrel, bladder, scandal, crossword, cough, talent, porthole

On cue, your blood pressure climbs, the brain obliged to work a little harder, because there's no clear logic behind the list. Thankfully all twelve are nouns at least—tactile for the most part—but that might be the sum of their connection. You could try clustering the list into sets of three or four, but a wiser approach is the narrative ploy.

Try weaving a story around the items, starting with a glove on a mattress. Better than a limp accessory, why not animate the glove to make it a ghostly hand beckoning you to enter your bedroom, gesturing hello from your queen-sized bed? Close your eyes and picture it. There, that's chalked in your short-term memory now, the so-called 'blackboard phase' of retaining facts.

Terrified by this ghostly glove, you run away down the hall, only to collide with a gigantic oyster that's blocking the way. An oyster?! Slowly,

the shell closes around you, a mollusc-version of an iron maiden, so you
drop to your knees and sing a psalm, the song's silent P sure to Piss off the
bivalve. Magically, this makes the oyster vanish, only for Sir Lancelot
to arrive from the bathroom, a squirrel juggling acorns on his lance.

You get the picture. Let one item link to the next, ensuring each prompt heightens the absurdity. The weirder the tale, the stickier the ingredients, the greater your recall of it is likely to be.

Another technique is called the memory palace. Romans knew the method as '*loci*', meaning 'places'—the technique of mentally planting data across a physical space you can easily recall. Let's return to your place, where that glove lived. Or possibly your front door, as we need to create a sequence to lodge the items as they appear, moving through your home as we gather the words, locus by locus.

As you approach your door, you see a glove dancing on your doormat,
the fingers like little legs. You pick it up and slip the glove on your hand
in the style of Michael Jackson, or a one-armed burglar. You step inside.
   Boing! *Who put this mattress on the floor? Oh well, the soft base*
makes it easier to sneak into your own home. And not just sneak, but
bounce—a bouncy burglar with one glove, kangarooing down the hall.

And so on, from hall to lounge to kitchen, or however your house is configured. Orators like Cicero built their own mental palaces in order to address crowds for hours without notes, reviving well-known buildings within their minds to curate a speech's key points, or sprinkling the bones of an argument around their internal forums.

The rationale behind such a method is twofold. Firstly, you integrate the new with the familiar, placing a 'porthole' in your laundry, or a 'scandal' in your linen cupboard. And secondly, you array the information into a sequence, a vital ploy for speechmakers who need to retrieve their points in order. So long as you have more than one palace in your repertoire: try using schools or offices, your local library, a bush track you can retrace. It's wise to gather an array of locations, otherwise your home will soon become a midden of miscellaneous mental junk from previous recollections.

Brain-wise, memory is stored via its own neural sequence. If you took the glove-and-mattress challenge a moment ago, those random nouns would now hover in your prefrontal cortex, the same bundle of neurons that Mike Pope suppressed while playing prone in the fMRI scanner. A large part of this lobe, when not dealing with decision-making or moderating social behaviour, is a virtual warehouse of input that needs retaining. The moment you meet a new group of people, say, and cop a litany of names to remember, your prefrontal cortex is on active duty.

Should you really have to remember these names—imagine you've just joined a new tour-group for a month—then that's when the hippocampus comes into play, a thoroughfare enlisted in the task of etching our memories more deeply via the entorhinal cortex, an electric bridge in the medial temporal lobe that links the hippocampus to the multiple folds of the cortex itself.

The hippocampus—Greek for 'seahorse', owing to the component's many twists and ridges—is responsible for encoding sensory experience (such as visual or auditory input) into new neural pathways, embedded for future reference. The names of our fellow travellers funnel from the forebrain, via the hippocampus, and into the depths of the temporal lobe. If used often while lodged here, this rollcall will soon enter the ranks of explicit memory, available in nanoseconds like the alphabet, for example, or the names of your family members.

But what happens when the hippocampus is missing? How does a brain cope when the ability to archive data is lost? Rather than speculate on that scenario, let's meet someone in that very situation: the world's most extraordinary puzzler, Henry Molaison, known to medical history as HM. (And hereafter known as Henry, since his family lifted his anonymity after his death in 2008.)

Crossword man

Childhood disease successfully treated by Salk vaccine (5)
Japanese capital to host 1964 Olympics (5)
Glass Menagerie *playwright who choked to death on a bottlecap* (9,8)

The clues represent a catalogue of geography and sport, plus medicine and literature. How did you fare? Even if you didn't know the cap of an eyedrop bottle undid Tennessee Williams, I daresay you knew his *Glass Menagerie*.

Likewise for Tokyo: most solvers could name Japan's capital without knowing its Olympic history. Maybe immunologist Jonas Salk has never crossed your radar, but polio is certainly sealed somewhere in your entorhinal cortex.

This delicate balance between known and unknown is the learner's constant mindset. Our brains carry established facts (the chemical symbol for iron, say) and must build on that bedrock as we learn compounds—extensions of that primary knowledge, adjusting to updates and more complex input.

Like few other people in history, Henry Molaison embodied that process. Born in Connecticut in 1926, some fifteen years after Tennessee Williams, Henry suffered epilepsy from an early age. While his seizures weren't constant, they were violent and growing more frequent, leading to Henry undergoing radical surgery when he was 27.

William Scoville at Hartford Hospital was the surgeon in charge. His was the scalpel to remove most of Henry's hippocampus, plus the core of both temporal lobes. Also culled were slices of the entorhinal cortex and the amygdala, the Greek 'walnut' that resides in the limbic system, storing many of our emotions.

The good news was that as a result of this surgery Henry was spared his epilepsy. The bad news: he now suffered anterograde amnesia. For the rest of his natural days, Henry was incapable of creating new memories.

The man could tie his shoes and make a bed, those mechanical tasks of procedural memory. He knew Shakespeare's first name, and could identify the boats you see in Venice. But he'd lost the ability to learn and remember new things. Worse, Henry struggled to imagine the future, since our concept of tomorrow is built on our record of yesterday.

Imagine I suggested we visit the local pool next Tuesday. You'd be able to recall the location of the pool itself, or pools in general, the reek of chlorine, the diving board. Whereas for someone like

Henry, a suggestion to visit the pool might only retrieve the colour blue. Or coldness on the skin. His present was paralysed, his future unimaginable. Yet there was some hope in the midst of Henry's plight, the very reason his limbo has become so widely studied.

On the surface of things, Henry had lost the capacity to learn, or even remember what he'd eaten three minutes ago. Yet, scratching deeper, there was something stranger going on, and the patient's new reality gave science a rare insight into how human brains acquire information.

It came down to word puzzles. Before going under the knife, Henry had loved doing crosswords, and he'd tackle at least two a day, establishing a robust archive of synonyms and antonyms within his memory, a trove of trivia and names, everything poised for explicit recall. And after his operation, the outpatient's ardour for puzzles only grew. Later in his post-operative life, he said, 'One thing I found out is that I fool around a lot with crossword puzzles. And well, it helps me in a way.' What's more, 'You have fun while doing [them] too.' No matter the time of day, Henry would rummage in the basket attached to his walker, pulling out the latest set of clues. He'd complete American-style quickies; most clues tested semantics or general knowledge, and Henry was capable of filling whole sections of the grid, if not the whole thing. He even coped well with advanced-level puzzles in a *New York Times* collection.

All up to a point, a very particular point in fact: he failed to register any event or celebrity, any film or neologism, postdating 1 September 1953, the day of his operation. The Rolling Stones were deaf to him. The Who was one big who? He had no grasp of Disneyland, Apollo 11, the Vietnam War. Henry lived, and solved puzzles, in the present while remaining exiled to the past.

Nonetheless, the crossword could well prove a conduit for new knowledge, or that was the theory Dr Brian Skotko was eager to test. Skotko, a clinical fellow in genetics at Boston's Children's Hospital, oversaw a series of trials with Henry, supplying him a series of custom-made crosswords. At its heart, the exercise was to measure the potential of gaining implicit memory—those details that subconsciously stick—via the agency of clues.

Skotko used clues like those which opened this section, each clue extending a pre-1953 fact—from polio to Tokyo—with an insinuated update. Would Henry glean the news via the clues? That was the question Skotko wished to examine.

Raymond Burr was a case in point. Before Henry's surgery, the American film actor had been well established, starring in such noir thrillers as *Desperate* (1947), *Pitfall* (1948) and *Abandoned* (1949). Yet since Henry's operation, Burr's greatest claim to fame had been his TV roles, including the title roles in *Perry Mason* (1957–1966) and *Ironside* (1967–1975).

Burr was a burr, therefore, a stubborn piece of knowledge snagged in Henry's temporal lobe. In memory, they are called anchor points; the grounded facts that underpin the subsequent developments. Burr was a name Henry knew, despite not knowing the new chapter of the actor's career, and apparently lacking the wherewithal to retain that update. But could a crossword teach him that new fact? What might be the impact of this kind of clue:

Perry Mason portrayer, Raymond (4)

Or:

He played TV detective Ironside, Burr (7)

Little by little, the bespoke puzzles introduced these elements into Henry's awareness. Frail links began in the man's neural map between the known and the new, the familiar and the updated.

John F. Kennedy was a further example. Before Henry's operation, the politician had already been prominent in the House of Representatives, becoming a senator in 1952. But that's where his career ended for the outpatient—Henry's post-op fog obscured Kennedy's rise to power. According to Henry, J.F.K. never became president, let alone being shot in Dallas in 1963. As for Jackie Onassis, the name meant nothing.

And yet, crossword therapy yielded results. While Henry floundered with remembering random numbers (despite being shown the same seven-digit sequence 25 times) or failed to crack a simple stylus maze presented on a screen, he did glean the twists in J.F.K.'s career. When

WHATDUNIT

In 2009, a team at Toronto University ran a comb over Dame Agatha Christie's eighty-plus crime novels. The project was led by Ian Lancashire and Graeme Hirst, doctors of English and computing respectively, using software to profile the author's overall text. And lying there, amid the arsenic and red herrings, they uncovered a lulu.

In her prime, Christie ruled detective fiction, generating over two billion sales. Quite apart from the intricate plots, her novels bristled with stylish syntax and a gimlet eye for detail. Yet those laurels slipped in her last fifteen books.

Typical was a latish work, *Elephants Can Remember*. The analysis revealed a sharp drop in word variety by almost a third in contrast to her earlier books, coupled with a significant climb in repeated phrases and indefinite nouns—like 'thing', 'something', 'anything'—as if the dame had lost her hold on language.

The plot of *Elephants* is equally telling: a senior crime novelist named Ariadne Oliver investigates a fishy murder–suicide from ten years earlier. The elephants of the title are the elderly friends of the dead, the unreliable witnesses strewn about the Cornish manses and nursing homes. Ms Oliver must separate truth from falsehood, fact from memory lapse. But she struggles, as does Dame Christie.

In fact, many critics perceive the novel's true villain as less the fictional murderer than dementia itself. The book shows how an embattled mind has fewer words to muster a growing number of loose ends. Christie was never diagnosed, but her threadbare later novels speak volumes about the writer's inner fugue.

asked if Kennedy was alive or dead, Henry responded that he had been assassinated. He later mentioned that Jackie Onassis was formerly Kennedy's wife, despite the marriage occurring two weeks after Henry lost his hippocampus.

President Bill Clinton on the other hand, the president at the time of Skotko's research, was un-stickable for Henry's mind. Devoid of an anchor point, the new name drew a blank, the intellectual links too soft to introduce the new leader.

Neuropsychologists call this the snowball effect, where the more you know, the easier it is to add knowledge. By design, crosswords accentuate this effect. On the first pass of the clues, you enter the answers you know. You jot down POLIO or PERRY MASON, each letter a potential anchor for the clues where the more elusive answers lie in hazier memory, the lesser known, or even the unknown. As Norman Doidge, the champion of neuroplasticity, writes, 'Experts don't store answers, but they do store key facts and strategies that help them get answers.'

Henry Molaison was less an expert than a creature of habit. He cracked the clues that seemed familiar, and then progressed as best he could from there, as we all do. Joe DiMaggio, the baseballer, was a household name for Henry, and ditto for Marilyn Monroe, their names linked in one encyclopaedic snowball. Yet the pair only married four months into Henry's post-op life; he learnt of it—or at least stumbled onto it—via crosswords. Thanks to these carefully constructed crossword clues, in tandem with the puzzle's intermesh, Henry collected several new titbits over three years of clinical puzzle-solving: he connected the Warsaw Pact of 1955 with World War II. He placed Raymond Burr on the television. He figured polio ('an illness . . . does something to the nerves') was cured.

But did any update linger? That was the fraught part to confirm for Skotko and Corkin. Once the information had arrived in HM's brain, would it stay?

Sadly, the answer seemed no. After Henry stopped solving the bespoke puzzles, pre-1953 reality returned in living colour, with next to no new information retained. J.F.K. never married Jackie, just as Joe never met Marilyn, and the Warsaw Pact dissolved.

Which illustrates another side of crosswording: as much as the hobby can gift you with facts or unfamiliar words, those same riches are only realised if you actively use them, and reuse them. If not carried from the prefrontal to the temporal lobe for safekeeping, the data you gain will likely fray from memory, like a glove forgotten on a bed. Like a mattress on which no impression remains. Care to recite those twelve random nouns I gave you to start this chapter? Don't tell me you've forgotten them.

The dementia dimension

Across Australia, over 425,000 people are living with dementia, as well as the million-plus people responsible for their care. Anguishing as the numbers are to read, the maths make it clear: if you aren't linked to a family member or loved one living with the condition, then you're the exception.

My own dad lived with frontotemporal dementia in his last seven years, shedding words in step with his volition as each year passed. Seeing first-hand this poignant reduction made me understand why most of us fret when forgetfulness strikes.

Not that such fears are always grounded. Forgetting is part of living. And the longer we live, the more there is to forget. Besides, there's forgetting a restaurant's name and drawing a complete blank about a recent event. There is forgetting the name of London's river versus the way home from the train station.

Joseph Jebelli, an English neuroscientist, and author of *In Pursuit of Memory*, puts it more plainly: 'Forgetting things in old age is not a sign of dementia. Your memory gets worse as it gets older, but that is fundamentally different from Alzheimer's.'

In the words of Henry Brodaty, the Professor of Psychogeriatrics at the University of New South Wales, 'We all become forgetful as we get older. We forget where we put the car-keys, or we forget people's names. But it's where loss of memory and other cognitive abilities lead to the interference in our daily lives that people cross a line, and say, "This is dementia."'

So the difference comes down to the lapse's gravity. Small things will slip our memory—that's only natural—but it's quite a different matter to forget how to cope. When it comes to symptoms that could signal dementia, significant memory loss is among a welter of other indicators, including severe mood changes, disorientation and problems performing familiar tasks. As a rule, doctors deem two or more such signs as being worthy of closer consultation.

Yet before we go further, let's clarify the language. Dementia is the umbrella term that includes Alzheimer's disease. As the name suggests, Alzheimer's is a disease and not a legacy of old age. When one is living with Alzheimer's, Jebelli explains, 'you're not losing your marbles, you have a serious illness', one that 'slowly takes away a person's autobiography'. Someone who loses their innermost memory loses themselves in many ways.

Other major forms of dementia are vascular (triggered by damage to the brain's blood vessels) and frontotemporal, as my dad underwent. Alzheimer's dementia is flagged by two key abnormalities in the brain. One is a build-up of amyloid plaque among the neurons, hindering their ability to fire. The second is a tangle within the neuron's cell body, chiefly from a structural protein called tau. The knottier it gets, the less efficient the brain's nutrient supply becomes.

Which brings us again to puzzles—and reading, and social engagement, and a dozen other activities thought to lower the risk of dementia. What faith can we place in criss-crossing words to keep dementia off the doorstep? Neuroscientists are in consensus: the practice of solving puzzles, while no magic shield against dementia, is unquestionably part of a healthy lifestyle that helps to safeguard your wellbeing into later life.

Cognitive neuroscientist Professor Keith Wesnes teaches at the University of Exeter. In 2017, he oversaw an online study of 17,000 healthy people in the 50-plus bracket. Volunteers tackled nine mental tests, from memory to reasoning. Once collated, the overall results revealed a strong trend.

For crossword fans, the news was bright. To quote Wesnes, 'Performance was consistently better in those who reported engaging in puzzles, and generally improved incrementally with the frequency of puzzle use.' While the fountain of youth has yet to be located, Wesnes added, 'Performing word puzzles was associated with an age-related reduction of around 10 years.'

Across the Atlantic, an equivalent study was held in 2012 at the University of California. The study recruited 65 healthy volunteers with an average age of 76, along with ten seniors living with Alzheimer's and ten people in their 20s and 30s. The entire cohort was assessed via a series of mental tasks, much like the Exeter study.

While it's worth noting this study's modest sample size, the Peter Pan effect of puzzling again emerged. This time around, the brains

HEALTHY HABITS

'Numerous studies,' reports Dementia Australia, 'suggest that engaging in more mentally stimulating activities through life is associated with better cognitive function, reduced cognitive decline and a lowered risk of developing dementia'. Aside from crosswords, and other puzzles such as sudoku, they recommend:

- reading in general
- listening to the radio
- visiting museums
- taking a course
- learning a new language
- eating a healthy diet
- engaging in regular exercise
- playing music and board games
- pursuing artistic and other hobbies
- participating generally in other social interactions.

of seniors who engaged in mentally stimulating activities, including puzzles, were comparable to those of the young people in the control group. By the same token, older volunteers without brain-bending habits scored results more aligned with those living with Alzheimer's.

So while we can't say a puzzle will cancel the risk of dementia, we can confirm a stream of regular crosswords can enhance your mental agility and reliable recall.

Perhaps the last word belongs to Miriam Raphael, contributor to a *Guardian* forum in 2016. The context was yet another cognitive survey conducted among seniors, this one issued by the Mayo Clinic in 2016, with crosswords counted as part of 'high midlife cognitive activity'. As readers debated the study's merits on the forum, Miriam chipped in: 'I'm just three weeks short of my ninetieth birthday, and both my husband and my neurologist have noticed some deterioration of my memory. But I still can solve crosswords, and I intend to continue to compete in crossword tournaments (and find my way home afterwards).'

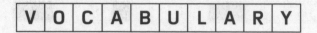

VOCABULARY

How porous is your thesaurus?

We are what we remember, our words included. So how many words do you know? Five thousand? Ten? Let me ask this another way: how many words have you met in your life, and retained? Vocabulary, after all, is a shorthand label for retrievable semantic memory.

This chapter plunges into the semantic, exploring how your cognitive health is reflected by the size and suppleness of your personal word-hoard, as vocabulary was once known. Along the way, we'll also summon puzzles and quizzes, seeing the role they play in verifying your known words, in addition to implanting the new.

So, again, how many words are listed in your mental Rolodex—twelve thousand? Fifteen thousand? Let's stick to English, to keep things simple. Or as simple as possible, since estimating which words your brain possesses is a special brand of folly. Where do you start? At A, of course, so: aardvark, aback, abacus, abalone, abandon.

But 'abandon' is the tip of the iceberg, because most words are part of a related bundle. 'Abandon' propagates 'abandoned' and 'abandoning', 'abandoner' and 'abandonment'. With one verb, you've inflated your vocab to five, which doesn't seem right. That's why linguists only count lemmas. If you don't know the term, let me advance your word-hoard by one. Greek for 'premise', *'lemma'* is a word adopted by the sciences, in particular mathematics where lemmas (or lemmata) are propositions proven on the way to testing further propositions. In linguistics, lemma applies to any headword in a dictionary, such as abandon versus its numerous offspring. Still, the mess remains, since where does a lemma start and an offshoot begin?

Wiser to defer to the dictionary, where any subsidiary word is listed within the headword's entry. Laugh, for instance, counts as a

READY, SET, COGITATE!

Below is a series of vocab chains, going from the familiar to the more arcane. How far along each sequence can you get until you strike a term that baffles? Definitions are below.

1. acumen—talisman—salacious—turpitude—prolix—zaftig
2. brio—limn—transom—martinet—sortilege—baldachin
3. despot—diurnal—vicissitude—lapidary—niqab—pandiculate
4. vestige—restive—redolent—louche—caesura—velleity

single word, waiving the need to tally laughter and laughed, laughing and laughingly, while laughing gas and laugh track count as separate headwords, each phrase its own distinct parcel of meaning and therefore valid as a word (or lemma, as you now know).

There, we have that much sorted. But when is a word a word? This paragraph has fifty-nine words, including the word fifty-nine, but do we include numbers in the final count? No, is the simple answer, although numbers are counted to a point, where four could denote a rowing team, a cricket boundary, a playing card, an early hour.

The next headache is wordworthiness, where words like rando for random, or murses for male nurses, feel too hokey to rate inclusion. Even now, trotting out wordworthiness only underlines how nonce words can still make sense, despite eluding the dictionary.

Quandary number four is polysemy, or multiple meanings. Brain the noun can become brain the verb, meaning to strike on the head. Many words carry this versatility. Count can be a noun, a verb, or a creep in Transylvania. Likewise skim can mean to read quickly, to flick pebbles across water, and scalp the cream off milk. Yet notice, in all three cases, a shallow and quick action is implied, deepening the dilemma of distinct meaning versus additional nuance.

Still, if you want some hardish numbers, then let's turn to Shakespeare. If anyone had a wealth of words, it was him. His works alone, from plays to sonnets, contain around 900,000 words in sum. Reduce that to unique words, and then down to lemmas, and the writer's vocabulary floated around 25,000, from the commonplace to the insufflated (full of air).

In modern terms, that's not a colossal sum, but still head-spinning. To quote British linguist David Crystal, 'No other author matches these impressive figures.' To quote Hamlet, 'Words, words, words.' To meet a few more words, and explore how vocabulary enriches your mind, let's go quizzing.

The basket in your head

Poilu is:
(a) French soldier
(b) taro paste
(c) facial hair
(d) bad poet

Acedia is:
(a) alien
(b) famine
(c) sloth
(d) refuge

Squill is:
(a) shriek
(b) sea onion
(c) tiny squid
(d) small shrimp

For the record, I scored two out of three. Poilu might be familiar to regular crossworders. Any short word ending in U is bound to be on high rotation. To that long-serving French soldier (an infantryman from World War I) you can add haiku, beau, lieu, ecru (yellowy-brown), coypu (beaver-like rodent) and, finally, adieu. Granted, you probably won't catch an ecru coypu, unless you happen to solve a stack of crosswords. Nor will a puzzle novice need to contemplate a poilu composing a haiku, yet that arcane litter is strewn across most solvers' greyscape like adhesive glitter.

As for acedia, the quiz's second word, I'd met that oddity early in my puzzle addiction, but not via clues in this case. Rather I'd met this synonym of sloth when reading the Collins Dictionary in 1988. ('Hello, my name's David and I'm a dictionary reader.') Recently, I returned to the notebook I'd kept at the time and upon seeing words like anlace and canephor, I failed to recall what they meant. They must have entered my short-term memory like murmurs, too faint for the hippocampus to register.

But acedia somehow stuck—and the reason lies in the pincer action of reading and solving. The obscure word entered my temporal lobe courtesy of a Gordius clue in *The Guardian* back in 2012:

Listlessness can make one reject help (6)

The clue's wordplay element entails ACE (*one*), then AID (*help*) *reject*ed to create DIA. Combined, the two pieces spell ACEDIA, a synonym of listlessness.

No cause for alarm if that clue makes scant sense at this point—we'll unpick the mechanics of cryptic language in Part Two. The clue's purpose here is to illustrate how crosswords, more than most language streams, are likely to summon esoteric words, much like 'esoteric'. One puzzle—cryptic or quick—can rummage the marginalia of a wider vocabulary, giving the passive words a gentle prod, reviving them in your memory for being summoned by the puzzle. Or, should the word be unfamiliar, the grid is there to help deliver it. With this playful repetition, a peripheral word can become a neural print, processed by the hippocampus into semantic memory, helping to fight the natural acedia of later years.

GRAIN BY GRAIN

The Free Rice Vocabulary Quiz <www.freerice.com> is a website combining brain food with real food for those in need. Visitors to the site can choose one of 60 levels of difficulty, from household words to out-there obscurities, including squill (that notorious sea-onion) on Level 57.

Your vocabulary is sure to grow, since whenever a word is missed, such as squill in my case, a subsequent quiz will return to the term, giving you a chance to snare the correct response. In so doing, you get to file the word in short-term memory, as well as guarantee the United Nations World Food Programme will be the richer for ten more grains of rice.

Squill, therefore, was my downfall. Before the earlier test, I'd never seen the word, not in crosswords or novels, not in research or conversation. I put that down to sea onions ranking poorly on the topical menu. Or any menu, since the bulbs are toxic, though Hippocrates did prize squill as a jaundice remedy. Perhaps now, with the Hippocrates curio working in tandem, squill may stick in the brain, leaving the blackboard mode of short-term memory for the realm of the declarative memory, or what facts and figures you have on call.

The mini-quiz is a foretaste of the Free Rice Vocabulary Quiz (see more details in the sidebar), the sort of test that does a lot to reinforce language and memory. In the same vein, there are quick crosswords too, each clue a means of accessing your word-hoard, each puzzle an informal inventory of the words you carry.

While quick clues don't tease the brain with inbuilt riddles, such as Gordius's ACEDIA clue, the style's crisscross diagram still allows for unfamiliar words to enmesh with the familiar. You fill in what you know, and letter-pattern helps you deduce what you don't, much as HM used anchor points to help intuit fresh input. So then, returning to the scenario of a stumped solver, a person in pursuit of a rare word meaning listlessness, the quick grid would offer a pattern like this:

_C_D_A

Consider these your anchor points, the key means of guidance that my clues in the fMRI tube had lacked. Though wherever you solve, your challenge is to exploit what you know to access what you don't. Here trial and error comes into play, your brain surmising what letters are likely to occupy the blanks.

Germans have a word for such cognition, as only Germans can. *Sprachgefühl* describes the intuitive feel one has for language, your sense of how words are constructed, and how they sit amid other words. The compound splices two nouns, where *Sprache* (language, or speech) accompanies *Gefühl* (feeling).

Juggle the possible suspects, from OCEDIA to ECUDIA—which aren't words—and soon your *Sprachgefühl* will settle on ACEDIA. A dictionary check will confirm your word-feel, assuming you're not too listless.

To enliven your own word-hoard I recommend the neural gym of crosswords—solve and stretch, solve and save. And whatever puzzles fail to provide, <www.freerice.com> can make up the shortfall, a site teeming with quizzes and quirkiness, from anlace (a two-edged dagger) to canephor (a sculpted figure carrying a basket on its head).

Homo lexicus

> *So when I was twelve years old, my mum said she wanted to talk to me about something. Um, my mum and I didn't have a lot of talks. I loved her very much but she was kind of an intimidating figure. She was one of those corporate working mums, with the beeper and the pantsuit and the rollie-suitcase. She yelled important things into phones a lot. And she was away a lot on business. But she sat me down in the living room and she told me that she was pregnant.*

Erin Barker, the twelve-year-old in question, is now in her 20s. She has a Masters in Creative Writing from the University of Southern Maine. She also has two trophies on her shelf, for twice winning The Moth's GrandSLAM storytelling competition with tales like the one above.

CROSSWORD-ESE—ODD WORDS THAT SOLVERS KNOW TOO WELL

Regular crossworders won't need to read the zoo plaques when encountering the okapi, the eland, the coypu or gnu. Ditto goes for the oryx or oribi. Nor will they miss a beat when meeting any of these frequent answers:

ADIT—mine's opening
AGA—Turkish official
AMAH—Indian nurse
ANOA—dwarf buffalo
APSE—church recess
ARETE—glacial ridge
ECLAT (and ELAN)—panache
ELVER—baby eel
ENNUI—malaise
ERATO—Greek muse
ERG—unit of energy
ETUDE—piano exercise
ETUI—sewing case

EWER—large pitcher
GUMBO—Cajun stew
IMAGO—adult insect
IMAM—Islamic leader
LIANA—jungle vine
LUAU—Hawaiian feast
OGEE—S-shaped moulding
OKRA—gumbo ingredient (see
   GUMBO)
POI—Polynesian staple
RANI—Indian queen
STOA—covered walkway
TOR—prominent crag

The Moth was hatched in New York City, back in 1997. Every few weeks, people gather in bars and clubs to tell stories on stage, drawing listeners closer to the light with their words.

Because that's the other dimension to vocabulary. More than a reckoning of the words you possess, vocabulary is also a hoard of connotation, a potential arsenal of rhetorical or emotional affect. This last section delves into that idea, meeting both clues and sentences to see what influence they confer on our brain.

Erin, the Moth champion, has a raconteur's flair—her voice is warm, her language disarming and her narratives pull you in. Thanks to those qualities, hers was the perfect material for a brain experiment at the University of California. A neuroscience team at Gallant Lab slid seven people into an fMRI scanner, wiring their skulls to monitors, as well as hooking up an audio feed of Moth stories. Alex Huth, the postdoc at the trial's helm, was hoping to see which segments of the brain recorded the greatest activity according to what words were being heard in which stories.

'The data we got in this language experiment were very complicated,' concedes Professor Jack Gallant, the lab's overseer. 'In fact, even our reviewers had a hard time wrapping their brains around it.' Because what they found was head-spinning, mind-bending. As the stories unfolded, the cortex twinkled. 'At the grossest level,' Gallant says, 'the experiment shows that each individual semantic concept, the meaning of each word, is represented in discrete brain locations, where each location represents a constellation of semantic concepts.'

Gallant uses the example of 'dog', the word. 'You know how a dog smells. You know how it looks, how it sounds when it barks. Maybe you had a dog bite you when you were a small child. And all that dog-related information will factor into your interpretation of the meaning of a story about a dog. All those brain areas associated with those different kinds of information will become activated to some extent.'

Dog, of course, is just one word. Erin Barker (no pun intended) has already uttered 90 in her opener, so imagine the carnival a listener's brain becomes upon hearing about her mum and that fateful conversation. Phrase by phrase—whether volunteers remembered their own mum, or maybe a disdain of loud phone-talkers—the disparate neurons responded to what they received, extracting fuel from the blood as each voxel (one of 50,000 volumetric units across the grey matter) was illuminated.

Apart from processing emotions, or dredging personal history, the brain can also play Dr Roget when receiving language, whether those words are heard or seen. Take a term like 'talk', say, which Erin uses in her opening sentence. In context, the word has a clear meaning. Here it denotes a private conversation between mother and daughter. There's no ambiguity. But that's not to say that versatile words with multiple meanings and shades don't rebound about the cerebrum until that sense is confirmed.

In fact, it seems likely that the brain categorises and subdivides words as they enter your consciousness, much like a librarian stacks their trolley according to the Dewey system.

Buoyed by the voxel patterns, Alex Huth and colleagues began to draft a brain atlas of language, a regional dictionary across the cortex. Although the experiment was not extensive, with only five men and two women monitored, making the atlas as much speculation as anything akin to a document of cadastral accuracy, the map was nonetheless fascinating. Huth arrayed colour-coded voxels into areas like Visual and Tactile, Outdoor and Body Parts, Time and Violence—a bubble-chart resembling a three-dimensional thesaurus.

It's intriguing to imagine running this same experiment to observe the brain of a puzzler at work. While a story like Erin's wields greater emotive clout than your average seek-a-word, there's no denying a bed of clues, or simple wordlist, has far greater lexical range than most stories can boast. In mainstream fiction, there are boundaries of word choices compared to a cryptic clue, which is a licence to pepper a solver's brain with no end of associations, the glossary unlimited, each clue a new context to decipher.

Like this treat from *The Times*, puzzle 10,972:

Club seals and we'd get hides (4,5)

Sorry, I know the image is bloody, but crosswords can confront your brain like that, emotive as much as deceptive. In one clue-set you can travel from Jane Austen to Austin, Texas, from acedia to Antarctica. If a Moth story can light up your brain, then a puzzle grid is liable to make the cerebrum dazzle.

The answer, by the way, has nothing to do with seal murder. This is called a hidden formula, where the solution is enfolded within the clue itself. Here the signpost for this ruse is *hides*, as in the clue *hides* the answer. The answer's definition, unrelated to seal leather or icecaps, is *club*. Look past the gore, the wallop, those innocent eyes, and you'll see the clue hides SAND WEDGE in consecutive letters, your missing club. And this is just a single clue among 36 in your average crossword, so the full set is bound to test your word-feeling as much as your feelings.

Hip-hip for the hippocampus

'Last week I got emphysema,' said the schoolgirl, 'followed by eczema and then psoriasis. After that, my teacher gave me antihistamines on top of hypodermics, which didn't really help because a few minutes later I ended up with anaphylaxis. I swear—that was the toughest spelling bee ever.'

Gotcha. That's the game jokes play, spinning a story to aim your focus one way, only for the punchline to subvert your perspective. Rather than ailing, the kid is spelling. Your relief prompts a laugh. In one phrase, reality flips, and your brain adjusts, plus or minus a smile.

That adjustment, that chuckle, is fundamental to this next chapter, where we gauge the effect humour has on our thinking, and how cryptic language can invert reality, and flip-flop outlooks with the best jokes in the playbook. The key to so many wisecracks, or cryptic clues, can be summarised by Mark Twain: 'Wit is the sudden marriage of ideas which before their union were not perceived to have any relation.'

Fresh links amuse the mind. Outsiders neglect that aspect when trying to grasp crosswords' appeal. They assume the attraction is solely aha, and never haha. Yet both matter—both reward the solver with the endorphin-rich joy of discovery.

Similar to jokes, the best clues conjure a scene in the mind. Here's a picture painted by Picaroon in *The Guardian*:

Fling with hunk is wild fantasy (7,8)

A solver may turn fifty shades of red, imagining rolling in the hay with their Fabio of choice, taking long walks on the beach. Yet this clue delivers a double happiness: the smile sparked by imagining this scene with the cognitive buzz of a breakthrough. Make *flingwithhunkis* go

PUNNET OF AMERICAN PUN-CLUES

The best US crosswords dabble in daffy definitions, where a word like NEIGH isn't just an equine utterance, but a 'Trigger warning?' (according to ace setter, Patrick Berry). How many puns can you undo below? The letter count and initial/s below will help.

1. Fleet runner? (7–A)
2. Old timer? (9–H)
3. Housecoat? (5–P)
4. Academic hanger-on? (6–T)
5. Losing proposition? (4–D)
6. One getting hit on at a party? (6–P)
7. Turning point? (3-2,4–UBD)
8. Where leopards are spotted? (6–S)
9. Nice one! (3–U)
10. Series with many numbers? (4–G)

ANSWERS: 1. admiral, **2.** hourglass, **3.** paint, **4.** tassel, **5.** diet, **6.** piñata, **7.** use-by date, **8.** safari, **9.** une, **10.** Glee

wild—as the wordplay is telling us—to spell WISHFUL THINKING, or fantasy.

We'll talk more about anagram recipes in the next section. For now this wild hunk is just a glimpse, to show how nimbly clues can jump from one train of thought to another, just as jokes can, warping the language's intent. There's one big difference, though: namely, jokes depend on a passive audience, while clues enlist your brain as accomplice.

To prove my point, let's meet a professor of English. The gentleman enters a pet shop, carrying a caged parrot. 'I'm sorry,' he says, 'but I need to return this bird as it uses improper language.'

The owner is surprised, since the parrot was in the shop for months and never once swore.

'Oh that's not it,' said the professor. 'Yesterday, the animal split an infinitive.'

Boom-tish—and you didn't have to flex a muscle or fire a neuron. Or maybe your brain tried to second-guess the punchline, putting the cells to greater work. All the hints were there, like Chekhov's pistol: why bother to specify the professor's field of study if that detail didn't pay off? Like anyone would, you probably assumed the parrot was a potty-mouth, the trope of countless jokes, and when that assumption collapses your surprise delivers the smile.

Psychologists call this incongruity, where an unseen outcome supplants the expected version. Whether the switch is passive (as in jokes) or active (as in Picaroon's fling), the promise of amusement is in the contract. Because laughter matters. For each guffaw, each titter and snicker, the cortex is awash with electric waves that have long fascinated neuroscientists.

When we laugh, the brain connects across the hemispheres. Even the amygdala, the temporal nub governing emotion, is swept into the hilarity. That's the peculiar bliss of laughter—the appeal of pealing if you like: as soon as we forfeit control, yielding to a mix of spasm and vocalisation, our brains sparkle from stem to stern.

Thanks to EEG recordings of a brain during laughter we know the anterior cingulate is prone to flare, that C-shaped network of neurons in the cortex's understorey, just millimetres above the right eye. This brain segment relates to reward and impulse, where the listener—or solver—sees the light.

Dr Dean Shibata, a professor in neuroradiology at the University of Washington, labels this internal lobe the brain's funny bone. When it ignites, the brain delights. When in stitches, the volunteers' adrenaline also abates, as well as their cortisol and norepinephrine, the fight-or-flight cocktail. Finally, a wicked giggle boosts endorphins, the natural joy drug in our central nervous system. All this confirms the platitude that laughter is medicinal.

This is cheering news, until you learn we laugh a modest fifteen to seventeen times a day, less than once an hour, according to a 1999 study conducted by two Ontario academics, Rod Martin and Nicholas Kuiper. So why so seldom? Since when did life get so solemn? And it needn't be the case, when you realise a cryptic clue can provoke more than a few grins. Going one better, a switcheroo clue can also reduce the animosity in your life. If you think I'm joking, read on.

Having words

He and I get into such rows! (8,5)

I love this clue, which hails from *The Times*, back in 2015. It makes me happy just to relive it—the deception so neat and solution so sweet that my brain smiles. Furthermore, it's a rare formula: the clue marries wordplay and definition into one happy union, despite the rancorous story it tells.

But before we solve this deception, let's explore a more surprising by-product of crossword solving, a dimension relating to rowing of the hostile kind, just as the clue suggests.

Harvard psychologist Christine Hooker supervised a study in 2010 to examine how couples resolve their differences. To qualify, couples needed to be in a relationship for longer than three months. Hooker then asked each person within the couple to keep an online journal over three weeks, recording any disagreements each participant had experienced with their partner.

This data was then measured against a lab test involving an fMRI reading and a string of photos. Each person in turn was shown pictures of their partner's face expressing a range of emotions, from happy to angry to neutral. The fMRI scanner registered the mental response the observers attached to each image. Across the cohort, male and female, the people to exhibit better emotional control were those whose brains showed stronger activity in the lateral prefrontal cortex.

As mentioned, this chamber is deemed the prime adjuster of our social behaviour. The same precinct is also vital to puzzle-solving, separating good from bad, as well as the knack of decision-making. Speaking to *The Telegraph*, Hooker went on to add, 'People who had a high lateral prefrontal cortex activity felt better [in the tests], and the people who had low activity continued to feel badly.'

WORDWIT

When I was young there were only 25 letters in the alphabet. Nobody knew why.

Never leave alphabet soup on the stove and then go out. It could spell disaster.

A teacher was telling her class about pronouns. She pointed to one boy, asking if he could give two examples. 'Who, me?'

I stayed up all night, trying to work out where the sun went. And then it dawned on me.

Twelve vowels, 23 consonants, a comma and a full-stop appeared in court. They are due to be sentenced next week.

Three intransitive verbs walk into a bar. They sit. They drink. They leave.

People who can't distinguish between etymology and entomology bug me in ways I cannot put into words.

Strange as it seems, partners who exercised their lateral prefrontal cortex more often had less capacity to harbour negative emotions. Such exercise included a regular dose of crossword-grappling, as Hooker's research found, whether the puzzles were attempted solo or as a pair. Testing your brain with twisted words, the study suggested, can readily lessen the chance of barbed words cutting too deeply. If your frontal lobe is habitually busy, then it's equally quick to process anger and disappointment, ensuring rows don't overstay their welcome. A crossword a day, you could say, keeps the animosity at bay. Or, resorting to the bumper sticker version: WORDS IN A ROW FORGIVE WORDS IN A ROW.

Which leads us back to that *Times* clue, the kind a couple might solve together and in so doing keep their rows to a minimum:

He and I get into such rows! (8,5)

The soap-opera scene is set: he yells at her (or him), just as the writer (I) bellows back. But stop. Remember the parrot who didn't swear and the schoolgirl who itched to spell 'psoriasis'. Go below the clue's surface and you'll find the punchline awaits. Because if you think the topic is a tiff, you've slipped. That's how the 'joke' is presenting, which should make you leery. Don't fall for the clue's misdirection—instead aim your focus another way, and soon the humour will dawn on you.

He is not a man, but He the noble gas that is Helium. And *I* is not the author, but Iodine, the stuff of antiseptics, possibly dabbed on psoriasis. As it happens, both pronouns are also chemical symbols, which align into atomic (not kitchen-sink) *rows* that comprise the PERIODIC TABLE. The gag, the laugh and the quarrel-easing pleasure is elementary.

Aaaah

Beyond a laugh, beyond a grudge repellent, a good puzzle also offers cranial pleasure for the solver, or a pair of solvers. Readers of *Puzzled*, one of my earlier books, may recall an email that served as proof of the erotic element to puzzling. The message came from someone known only as Alamala, who wrote to Radio National on hearing my broadcast about puzzle-making:

> *I am one of a couple of cruciverbalists—that's couple, as in two people, who snuggle up together over cryptic crosswords. We're evenly matched and complementary in that we have different areas of specialist interest. The satisfaction of this shared and cooperative intellectual activity brings us closer and excites our bodies via our minds. Usually we manage to finish at one go, but sometimes pen and puzzle are set aside for a more urgent activity . . .*

The jury has spoken. Cranial pleasure can invite the carnal too, with crosswords ticking three boxes in one—the aha, the haha and the aaaah as well.

Exhibit B for such a claim is a query from a *Herald* reader called Alice Cairns: 'I'm looking for a word which names the joy you feel when discovering that the answer you've managed to derive from the clue is in fact correct, albeit a word you've never heard of. Is there such a word?' The obvious suspect is serendipity, the act of discovery via happy accident. But that wasn't quite right.

I looked to German as a likely saviour, just as *Sprachgefühl* had furnished the language gap in the previous chapter. Salvation however came in the shape of phony German, more specifically a glossary compiled by English humorist Ben Schott by the name of *Schottenfreude: German words for the human condition*. This bogus A–Z includes such gems as *Einsiedelei* (the melancholy of cooking for one) and *Ringrichterscham* (embarrassment at being present when a couple argue). Between both terms lay *Irrleuchtung*: the surge of pleasure you experience as you solve a crossword clue. Was this the answer English lacked?

In the end I turned to social media, sharing Alice's question to the Twittersphere, causing an avalanche of replies. It's safe to say that every solver knows this unique brand of happiness, just as every solver has their own label for the sensation. Suggestions ranged from 'logofelicity' to 'smilitude'. Others plumped for 'crossguessing' or 'fulfillment', or, the more ersatz German of *Vermutenfreude* (suspicion-joy). But the showstopper came from an ex-journo called Zena Yeoh Armstrong, her tweet ending all arguments: 'The word you want is orguessm. I experience this feeling at least once every Friday.'

Eureka. The puzzle was solved. The brain could relax, or the body shake in laughter, as crosswords once more delivered their signature magic: *aha, haha, aaaah*.

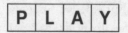

Survival of the funnest

When I say play, what comes to mind? Actors on a stage, perhaps, or the swish of a cricket bat? Puzzles in a magazine, maybe, or mahjong tiles in a box? Play could be the button on your remote—the arrow that starts the show—or playing in the musical sense. Or play can be what kids do, dragging out the Lego, the textas, the dress-up box. Thinking in binary mode, play could be seen as work's opposite, something you squeeze into a weekend, the R&R that lightens the 9-to-5 load. Playing with the notion of play, this chapter shall explore mischief of the cognitive kind, proposing that play is more a state of mind. Even the game we're playing now, bending play in multiple directions, is the rubbery thinking to counter a more concrete outlook—a cerebral version of elastics to see how far any notion can stretch.

The linguistic origin of the word is uncertain: there's the Dutch *'pleien'*, meaning 'to rejoice, or dance' or *'plegan'* in Old English, meaning 'to move rapidly, to busy oneself'. Whatever its roots, play is a catch-all term—take any tangent, you can't go wrong. Shakespeare used the word 422 times across his 37 plays, from roleplay ('Let me play the fool') to gameplay ('If thou dost play with him at any game'), with a dozen nuances in between.

Yet play is viewed indulgently by many adults—something frivolous, the antonym of earning your keep. 'Child's play' is facile by virtue of idiom. Exasperated parents tell their noisy darlings to go away and play—play whatever, it doesn't matter. It's make-believe, inconsequential.

But we must guard against that mindset. The more we limit our notions of play, the poorer we become. According to Arnold Toynbee, the English historian, 'The supreme accomplishment is to blur the line between work and play.'

Shrewd advice, should you ask Pat Kane, a futurist from Glasgow, and author of *The Play Ethic*. To Kane, play is all about adaptability and potential. A play theorist and consultant, Kane defines play as 'taking reality lightly'—the antidote to routine and competition. 'Ever since the Reformation,' says Kane, 'puritans have been telling us that play is at best trivial, at worst demonic and the very least not work.'

According to Kane, the play mode is 'boundary-challenging, reality-defying, insanely optimistic and relentlessly experimental,' because when children lack the rules they'll invent them. Play is less a game than *being* game, daring to surrender to the imagination. A young kid will talk off-script or fall into silence, engaging their mind in the all-encompassing now. Subsumed in play, a child adapts and imagines, tests or obeys their whims, sees where new pathways lead. All the while, as play unfurls, the player will believe in what they are doing, even if it's make-believe.

In maturing, for want of a better word, we lose touch with that mind-frame. German philosopher Friedrich Nietzsche underscored the challenge: 'The struggle of maturity is to recover the seriousness of the child at play.' As puzzle-maker and writer, that quote is my cornerstone. Rather than play, the quote's crux is seriousness, purely because it doesn't seem to belong. Surely play embodies fun, right? The pastime is an amusement after all—so why so serious?

The answer becomes clear whenever an adult joins a child at play. Believe me, if you've ever tried, you're likely to be assigned one of two roles: the monster—the play's enemy and ogrish threat from beyond—or the underling, play's apprentice. The reason why is trust, or lack of it. Adults can't be peers. Unless we surrender our status, we can't be seen as truly belonging to play, since we don't treat play seriously enough. Play should find us at our most plastic, and not in that hard-baked Lego kind of way. Mind you, away from the kits and manuals, Lego involves the shedding of rigidity, where play can lead to infinite outcomes, a slew of inventions and creations.

So where does play stand in relation to puzzles? By rights a puzzle seems more controlled than your typical spell of Lego. Clues demand a single answer, in meaning and length, with very little wiggle room.

Does that mean puzzle play is more of this adult limitation? To a large extent, the answer's yes. One clue awaits one answer, after all: the very definition of prescription. Yet cryptic play elicits far more than a single outcome as this chapter will reveal, the playful mindset a vital element in helping a solver reach that elusive eureka.

To see this truth played out, let's consider play in the sense of 'give', like the so-called give of a slack rope, a margin of leeway, a looseness of thinking that characterises play. When solving puzzles, the brain can't afford to be reductive in its thinking. Focus and logic will often yield rewards, but so does wiggle room, bringing an element of give to your thoughts. Canny solvers can play loose with a clue's potential meaning. Success will often rest in the art of imagining other answers, lying in other directions, rather than obsessing over one interpretation, with one result.

Failure by the same token can also lie in wait, thanks to considering a word or clue from multiple directions. Blue, say, could denote the colour, or a fight, or a risqué synonym, just as the word may signal the sea, the sky, or serve as a substitute for gloomy. Not every tack will be the right path. That's the nature of playful thinking: testing ideas, and learning from dead-ends rather than dwelling on those decisions as failures. My time in the tube, after all, saw my brain miss some 40 per cent of the clues, as much a symptom of pursuing false paths in the short time allocated as genuine bewilderment overall.

Indeed, there's a danger in seeing a clue one way, and no other way. Lapsing into that groove, you anticipate the look and shape of the answer before you get there, as if your next matchstick puzzle has a solitary way to be viewed, and thus one solution to be fetched.

Instead of life, the novelist Henry Miller might well have been describing puzzles when he said, 'One's destination is never a place but rather a new way of looking at things.'

The maxim underpins the puzzler's mindset, the give you need to find the way home, toying with the puzzle.

The same words echo the pleasure principle that many solvers know, the reason why puzzles are classified as play in the first place. Don't we all crave new ways to see things? Neuroscientist David Eagleman talks about the human trait of repetition suppression, that hunger we feel to experience the new, the joy we derive in the novel. That joy, in a sense, is also bundled into play, as our next section illustrates.

Loving solving

Time to visit the University of Buckingham, where two psychologists, doctors Kathryn Friedlander and Philip Fine, put 805 crossword solvers through their paces in 2015. The world-first experiment sought to understand what drives and distinguishes the sharper solvers of cryptic crosswords—their overall capacity to analyse and outwit the setter's wiles. The study was also geared to ascertain their backgrounds, motivations, levels of education and careers. While most of the group hailed from Great Britain, there was a reasonable smatter from the United States, Australia, New Zealand and India, among five other countries.

Solving prowess was also considered, the volunteers divided into three categories of competency:

Ordinary—solvers who (by self-report) normally take longer than 30 minutes to solve quality broadsheet cryptics, such as *The Times* or *Guardian*, mastheads with a reputation for more guileful clues—as soon to be seen in the many sample clues of Part Two. The same solvers don't usually tackle advanced cryptics, where a complex theme may govern the grid, or influence the answers in some way. And if they do, their success is limited.

Experts—those who can routinely solve one quality broadsheet cryptic in 30 minutes or less, who may compile crosswords professionally, or who tackle those more advanced, thematic cryptics with regular success.

Super—people who edit or compose cryptics professionally, on at least an occasional basis, for broadsheet or specialist publications; or those who regularly speed-solve a cryptic in under 15 minutes; or those who'd cracked tough puzzles consistently, such as the notorious *Listener* puzzles, with their barred diagrams, arcane vocabulary and rule-pushing motifs.

Never had such a herd of guinea pigs been mustered. The study lent science a rare chance to meet the puzzle page's consumer, so to speak, and several intriguing patterns emerged. As Dr Friedlander revealed, 'We found solvers tended to be qualified in scientific fields such as maths, computing, chemistry and medicine. What's more, this trend increased significantly with expertise.'

Sure enough, among the super solvers, roughly a third worked in IT, compared to just a fifth within the ordinary group. Word power, in other words, was just one aspect of the study. If the data was any yardstick, the best brains also relied on logic and an appetite for code-cracking.

This inference was supported in the study's own RIASEC survey, a model enabling the researchers to profile each solver according to their cognitive makeup. Also dubbed the Holland Codes, after US psychologist John Holland, RIASEC is a survey-derived glimpse into how different brains operate. The acronym stands for:

Realistic—the doers, the pragmatists, the DIY-ers
Investigative—the thinkers, from scientists to software developers
Artistic—the creators, the innovators, the designers
Social—the helpers, the teachers, the caring professions
Enterprising—the persuaders, the broadcasters, the sellers
Conventional—the organisers, the managers, the archivists

Looking at the list above, can you guess which two brain-modes were more prevalent across the Buckingham study, the two traits most shared by the solving elite?

Turns out the crossword gang displayed a strong Investigative mindset (over 40 per cent bias versus the typical 10 per cent among American solvers, according to an equivalent US study), as well as rating A for Artistic. In this category, the cryptic solvers reached the teens in most cases compared to 2 per cent in the general US pool.

The appetite to solve was another revelation. When it comes to tackling cryptic crosswords, Friedlander suggested, 'The ability to think flexibly seems more important than hours of practice.' Indeed, practice fell second to the desire to engage, going by the survey responses.

ALPHAGRAMS

Here are twelve possible Scrabble racks, each one holding at least two bingos (words using all seven tiles). As an added vocabulary test, one bingo is common, the other less familiar. AADEIRT, for example, yields RADIATE but also TIARAED and AIRDATE.

1. AAINRST	5. AEEFIRS	9. AEGNORS
2. ADEGNRT	6. AEEIMRT	10. AEHILNR
3. ADEIILS	7. AEELNST	11. AEIMNOR
4. ADEIOTS	8. AEENRTV	12. AEIMNRT

ANSWERS: 1. ARTISAN, TSARINA, **2.** GRANTED, DRAGNET, **3.** DAILIES, LIAISED, **4.** TOADIES, IODATES, **5.** FREESIA, FAERIES, **6.** MEATIER, EMIRATE, **7.** LEANEST, LATEENS (sails), **8.** VETERAN, NERVATE, **9.** ORANGES, ONAGERS (wild asses), **10.** INHALER, HERNIAL, **11.** ROMAINE, MORAINE (glacial debris), **12.** MINARET, RAIMENT (apparel)

'Many people . . . might be surprised at how little deliberate practice is done when it comes to crosswords. Solvers really don't hone individual components of cryptic crosswords (such as anagrams) in the same way as chess players learn opening gambits, Scrabble players learn alphagrams, and violin players practice scales.'

Alphagrams, for non-Scrabble zealots, are seven-tile clusters that the best players memorise (see the box above). CELRSTU, for example, is the alphagram of CLUSTER, just as AELOSTZ is the alphagram of ZEALOTS. Embed these sequences into your brain, where each cluster's aligned in alphabetical order, and the neurons might salvage that crucial bingo, a seven-tile play, at the next tournament. The logic behind the ploy is to allow any letter-string to resonate as soon as the pro-Scrabbler arranges their tiles from A to Z.

Crossword solvers are made of different stuff. Feedback from Buckingham reveals the elite rely more on the urge to solve, to bug the brain, rather than any notion of rehearsal or self-betterment. The name of the game is play, in other words. With few trophies or no salary to claim, cracking a puzzle serves as its own reward. 'The solvers have a drive to think,' Dr Friedlander observed. 'An itchy brain they need to scratch whether in their hobbies or in their challenging careers.'

Crosswords embody a duel with the setter, an agile sport for two minds where the playspace is the alphabet. Another analogy that solvers invoke is a treasure hunt, the seeker's brain roaming the grid in hope of the PDM (the penny-drop moment, to quote the study)—that wonderful flare in the frontal lobe. What few rules there are serve as a compact between code-maker and code-breaker, a protocol to encourage wide-open thinking, where any word could murmur an allusion, if your mind is alert enough to hear it. Come the endgame, the final clue unravelled, and the last answer lodged in place, the solver's urge to play (and replay) is only whetted.

D I S / C O N N E C T

Time to break and remake

Can you connect tennis to fish? It's not easy, I'll give you that—the two ideas seem at odds. One is a game played by humans, the stuff of Wimbledon and Rebound Ace, while fish, well, swim in rivers and other places where tennis is hard to play. Keep pushing however, keep telling your brain a link exists, and you may just find one. Or several. Andy Murray, for instance, has a river for a surname, the same name ending with ray, a fish. Then there's Pat Rafter—another surname suggesting rivers—who set up tennis schools across Australia, and fish are also found in schools. Tennis players need lines, a net, much like fishermen. And back in the noughties, a lanky right-hander named Mardy Fish ranked in the world's top 100.

Approaching the problem from the other direction—trying to build a bridge between fish and tennis—we can make all kinds of leaps. To fish is to angle, and tennis is a game of angles. Then you have scales, precisely what the ranking system does, scaling the jackpot pool for the bigger fish in the pond, the Novaks and Serenas, all the way down to the minnows. And lastly there's Pat Cash in his heyday—that chequered headband trying to control a 12-inch mullet.

So what? What's the big deal if fish and tennis share a few overlaps? The world has bigger problems to fry. But I disagree. Few challenges in life toss you into the weird mode of thought, called 'dissonance' in clinical circles, where the brain seeks to reconcile the conflict of separate ideas.

This chapter will explore several surprising links between puzzles and agile thinking, probing an area that many cognition books overlook, namely the business of tying together, and untying. Of tasking your brain to fuse two notions as nimbly as the same puzzles oblige you to un-fuse them. To solve a cryptic clue in particular, you must refuse the lazy associations, and instead unlink and make new connections.

The practice is vital in multiple fields, from engineering to medicine, from art to IT, pursuits far removed from the puzzle page. Indeed, the history of invention is a tribute to fresh connections. Mentally, Philo Farnsworth leapt from a ploughed hill to the dissected field of cathode emissions, making way for the TV screen he'd create. Adolf Fick, a German GP, imagined the meniscus from an ear of corn as a concave cap for the cornea, thus designing the contact lens.

As it happened, my own corneas were focused on Farnsworth's telly when the tennis/fish dissonance landed on my lap. I was watching the Paris Open final in 2010, where Sam Stosur the Australian was playing the tournament's seventeenth seed, Francesca Schiavone. Out of habit, I was barracking for the Aussie, but the Queenslander was being outsmarted, out-thought and out-angled by her Milanese rival. Initially I felt deflated, watching my compatriot flounder (hey, there's another fishy link), until I saw the bright side.

The answer lay in SCHIAVONE, the surname. Can you see the fish in those letters? Why not release them into a random shoal?

$$H \quad A \qquad E$$
$$C \qquad O \qquad\quad S$$
$$I \qquad N \quad V$$

Sitting on the couch, trying to stay awake, I spun the letters in my head and chanced on something succulent. I say chanced, but Louis Pasteur, another scientist and inventor was more of the opinion that, 'Chance favours the prepared mind.' In truth, my brain tackles these quirks all the time, finding anagrams and other curiosities in names and phrases. Like a tennis player's forearm, my noggin is stronger for alphabetic drills as well as a craving to find connections. This is due to puzzles obliging the brain to build bridges between unlikely banks. It destroys bridges too, but let's keep things constructive for the moment.

Have you netted the hidden fish? I refer to ANCHOVIES, those nine letters ready-made to occupy a crossword grid, so long as Schiavone could outlast Stosur in the final. That way, the Italian was assured sufficient fame to qualify for an anagram clue, assuming I could link the clue's two domains—tennis and the ocean—in the subsequent clue.

If that makes no sense, let me explain. A core principle of crossword-setting is akin to marriage, unifying a clue's two parts—the wordplay and the definition, or vice versa—so snugly you can't detect the line of separation. Very soon Part Two will unlock the mechanics of cryptic puzzles in greater detail. For now, let's just consider Schiavone as a perfect red herring, a scrap of mental bait that I could use to make an anagram clue, so long as I could match the tennis player (her name the letters you had to mix) with something fishy (the definition pointing to ANCHOVIES, the solution).

Drafting the puzzle, I tried to splice those elements into a fluent entity, that had my solvers thinking tennis (the wrong, lazy connection), and overlooking fish (the right one). To make that deception possible, I had to build a bridge in my own mind. With ANCHOVIES, the answer, I needed a tennis-y image to echo fish, or a fishy notion evoking tennis. Do this right and both parts would seem one unbreakable unit, leaving my solver at sea, unsure how to disjoin the elements. Something like this:

Net catches these Schiavone smashes (9)

Spot the trap? Talking all things tennis, I'm nudging your gaze one way, towards the court heroics in Paris, when really you should be pondering the sea. The craft is called misdirection, getting a solver's brain to make a false association.

For the same reason, 'cryptic' the word derives from '*kryptos*' in Greek, or 'hidden'. Every puzzle, every clue, compels a solver to go seeking, if you like—to expose the phony link and forge the hidden one.

With this clue, you need to recognise Schiavone as a letter cluster, not a tennis player. You need to smash those letters—S, C, H, I, A, V, O, N and E—and next align your result to the ambiguous net that opens the clue.

That's the cryptic art in a nutshell, for both setter and solver. The setter builds a diversion out of sly connections, while the solver's challenge is twofold: to fracture the lie and then reconcile the two parts to reveal the answer. Call it a binary way of staying brainy.

CELEBRITY COCKTAILS

If SCHIAVONE hides ANCHOVIES, can you swirl the ten complete names here to make a single word each time? (The clue is in the brackets.) AL GORE, say, gives you GALORE or GAOLER—while PRESBYTERIANS congregate in BRITNEY SPEARS.

1. MEG RYAN (Eurozone?)
2. SOCRATES (Rudest or roughest)
3. MONA LISA (East African)
4. STEVE IRWIN (Q-and-As)
5. NICK PRICE (Alfresco feaster)
6. NOVA PERIS (Oozing through)
7. RED SYMONS (Medical conditions)
8. FATS WALLER (Cascades)
9. ISAAC STERN (Verifies)
10. BEN COUSINS (Boing-boing . . . ?)

ANSWERS: 1. Germany, **2.** coarsest (plus coasters), **3.** Somalian, **4.** interviews, **5.** picnicker, **6.** pervasion, **7.** syndromes, **8.** waterfalls, **9.** ascertains, **10.** bounciness

That's the buzz of crosswording, for both parties. But how will your brain conduct such contrary work—breaking and remaking? And what's the net benefit of this whole fishy racket? Read on.

The art of re-seeing

Your brain knows how to apply the word 'apply'. The verb crops up in legal clauses and shampoo labels all the time. The root is Latin, linking back to '*applicare*', meaning 'to connect'. Going one step further back, the stem is '*plicare*', meaning 'to fold', giving us such cousins as ply and pliant, imply and complicated. Of course, you know all these words and how to use them, each stored in the folds of your brain.

But now look at the word again. Apply. Can you see the word from a different perspective? Look again, carefully:

Apply

A hint: consider a woman called Maria Ann Smith. She came to Australia in 1838, travelling from England to settle in outer Sydney. There she established an orchard where the first shoots of a promising new plant germinated, a green fruit that would soon bear her nickname: Granny Smith.

Apply. Do you now see the word anew?

Odds are the pioneer yarn has jolted your frame of reference. In a flash the familiar turns fresh, the 'apply' of legal clauses now a descriptor of Jonathans. If zest is lemony, why can't a turnover be apply?

Linguist Geoffrey Pullum calls this category of word a 'misle', a playful backformation of 'misled'. Coworkers, for instance, could be seen as those responsible for orking cows, the word allowing your brain to enter a new interpretation. Mothers in a different light could be insect collectors. Superbowl might describe an excellent hooter.

It's all total nonsense, yet there's a logic behind the gaffes, just as warbling might be deemed military medals, while misled rhymes with fizzled. Working with language in orthodox ways makes for orthodox brains. Muscles betray our lifestyle—from the oversized calves of the cyclist to the beer-lover's paunch. In the same vein, our brains reflect our dominant mode of thinking.

Let's meet Dr Debra Aarons, an academic at the University of New South Wales. Aarons specialises in generative grammar, a branch of linguistics that regards grammar as a mental system of rules that generates an infinite number of sentences. Pioneered by Noam Chomsky, generative grammar labels our inbuilt ability to process language as tacit knowledge of grammar. As infants, even before we can read we learn to grasp simple and compound sentences, understand the various parts of speech and the working rules of case and tense. Immersed in language, we cotton on to grammar long before we know the word itself.

But if we stick to that diet, neglecting to learn additional alternative languages—be they cryptic or Portuguese—our brain gets lazy. Neural pathways channel the same old traffic, and our input becomes as predictable as our cognitive responses.

In 2015, Aarons decided to examine this mindset. As part of her puzzle-flavoured paper called 'Following orders', the linguist investigated the impact of cryptic clues on mental pliancy. Clue by clue, the paper examined numerous cryptic formulas, and how they might influence our inner wiring. Rather than brain-mapping, or resorting to fMRI scanners, Aarons unpacked each recipe to test how their ludic—or playful—nature could spur the mind to process language in a different way.

We've already dabbled with anagrams, getting the neurons to juggle a tennis star into a pizza topping. But what about charade clues, wondered Aarons, a recipe that dismantles an answer into fragments. HEART, say, can be split into HE-ART, or possible HEAR-T, since single letters can also be detached. Answers to Aarons' charade clues, from BALL-A-DEER to DI-SCOUR-AGE, show how the breakdowns preserve the whimsy of Pullum's misles.

PENCHANT was another specimen cited by Dr Aarons, warranting the clue:

Oinking tendency?

Pigs oink. And pigs live in sties, also known as pens. Therefore a pen-chant could be viewed as oinking, or a chant escaping a pen.

Cheap trickery, you might argue, but Aarons has a different take: 'In viewing language elements as pieces to be joined without regard for rules of linguistic structure and use, cryptic crosswords force solvers to work against their grammatical intuitions.' Push hard enough, dismantle far enough, and fresh cognition will come: 'Once we view language, especially written language, as a string of elements, the play and puzzle possibilities are endless.'

Thanks to cryptic language, or the warbling whimsy of misles, a word like penchant converts into an ambiguity your mind must decipher. Is heart an organ, say, or a reference to machismo paintings, the he-art your eye can also detect? Is sewer a drain or a seamstress? Equipped with a new way of thinking, your brain is obliged to play a momentary tug-of-war with itself, trying to rationalise the mixed signals on offer.

To appreciate that tension in the visual realm, look at the Necker cube below, an elegant mind-trap designed in 1832. With no orientation cues, your brain must determine whether A or B is closer to you.

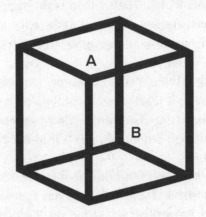

Naturally the answer is either, depending on how you view the cube. Should you feel A is nearer, this would place that letter in the downward-pointing outer corner. Likewise, if you picked B as closer, that letter would occupy the upward-pointing outer corner, essentially flipping the cube in your mind's eye.

The Necker cube is a shape-shifting paradox, realigning your neural path just as 'penchant', 'mothers' and 'coworkers' can be linguistic illusions, coaxing your brain to see two truths. Like Necker's cube, only one orientation can be perceived in any given instant, a fleeting reality quickly disrupted by the alternative, and vice versa.

Whether visual or verbal, the bottom line is cognitive. Your brain can't rely on tacit grammar any more than it can trust orthodox perceptions. Not all the time. The gist is dissonance, the constant flux of competing signals, where ovaries can mean eggs, or a coded description of monotony, yet never both at once. Optical illusions, like cryptic mischief, force the mind to flicker, to juggle and arbitrate, rather than doze in the usual monotony. As adults we deal with pragmatics—the rules of grammar, the roles of words—but with the cryptic 'modality' we can abandon the script.

Try Vlad's clue from *The Guardian*:

Old police force's making arrest (6)

The clue smoothly persuades you to think of law and order. Yet don't be misled. Remember the tennis example. Change from a reader to a solver and decide where to disconnect the sentence.

Despite its judicial vibe, Vlad's clue is more concerned with physics than civics. Not just a legal term, arrest is also a verb familiar to scientists when measuring momentum. Cast your mind back to your own days in your high-school lab, going through Newton's laws of motion . . .

Or approach the answer from the opposite side. That's a general tip for solving: if one end isn't revealing the solution, try the other. Just as Necker's cube can be reorientated, so too can a cryptic clue, this time by placing the old police force in the foreground. Does any old force spring to mind? Like 'arrest', 'force' can be a scientific term, but here the judicial context is the right one: we are indeed seeking a vintage cop squad, or maybe the force still exists. Who could tell? This force is secretive after all . . .

For the answer I suggest you travel back to Germany, when the wall was up and paranoia reigned in Berlin. The force's official name was/is the *Ministerium für Staatssicherheit*. Not that Vlad expects you to know that, but most solvers will recognise the service's abbreviation, 'Stasi'.

Almost there. Keep pushing. There's one more connection to make.

No matter the genre, quick or cryptic, a crossword solution must mirror the case of the clue's definition. Here in Vlad's case the apostrophe does that duty, contracting the expression to read: *old police force's*. STASI, therefore, isn't your answer, since you too must mimic the clue's grammar, converting the secret police into STASI'S. And look, the minute you close that gap, the cops disappear, morphing into STASIS, a synonym of arrest, but less in the cop sense, and more to do with monotony.

MISLEADING MISLES

Biped—past participle of bipe
Bookings—deplore royalty
Codify—to convert into a cod
Epitome—a large epi-pen manual
Menswear—they sure do
Nowhere—and later, somewhere else?
Persephone—mobile unto itself
Pronouncement—the stuff that keeps you and I together
Putin—enter
Repaired—reunited
Sabotage—the era of wooden shoes
Tumbling—navel piercing
Unionised—amalgamated into a union
Weeknights—Camelot tots

To quote Dr Aarons, 'When working with language as bits of code, puzzlers are thrown constantly onto their linguistic intuitions, and consciously have to fight against them.'

There's the gauntlet at your feet: to unlock a cryptic puzzle, you need to foster a second instinct, to imagine the alternative and see the covert: just the sort of thinking that leads to the laboratory. And by laboratory, of course, I don't mean lab-oratory.

Super solutions

There are inventions anywhere you look—from parachutes to pulsars, from GPS to DNA—with backstories vouching for the benefit of a brain leaping sideways. Look at books, say. We take them for granted, yet we owe their existence entirely to an inspired reverie in 1439, when a German silversmith named Johannes Gutenberg called by a vineyard. There he saw a large-scale wine press squashing grapes into juice, the fruit stomped flat between two metal plates—and he made a connection. *What if,* thought Gutenberg. *What if you placed blocks of movable type along the lower plate? What if instead of grape juice there was ink?*

Edward de Bono would label Gutenberg's insight as a classic instance of lateral thinking. De Bono coined that phrase during the 1960s to describe a creative and indirect mode of problem-solving. We see it every time someone finds a novel use for an object, like a bush mechanic's repair job, cutlery as jewellery, or the rebirth of tyres as flip-flops in Nigeria.

In a sense, our own brain flips, linking two ideas to forge one neat solution. Say you're stuck in a hotel room with no iron for your shirt. A crafty guest might heat the room's frying pan and improvise with its base. Don't imagine that an iron, and only an iron, is the unique answer to your problem—that's the trap of one-track thinking. Lacking X, a limited thinker will treat X as the single remedy.

Another trap, as de Bono has identified across his suite of 'thinking' titles, is the notion that any creative idea is logical in hindsight. When Gutenberg saw the grapes and visualised type-blocks, he was being creative—not logical. Of course, as you flick the pages of this book, or watch galley proofs rolling from a press, everything seems logical, where wineries paved the road for libraries as though it has always been. But that impression neglects the fact that most breakthrough solutions are the fruit of flexible minds.

Science journalist Steven Johnson calls it the 'adjacent possible'. Described as an inventive mindset, the adjacent possible 'captures both the limits and the creative potential of change and innovation'. In his book, *Where Good Ideas Come From,* Johnson typifies this tinkering approach as 'hovering on the edges of the present state of things, a map of all the ways in which the present can reinvent itself'. Instead of being mired in the present—the room with no iron, the grid with no answer—the nimble thinker ponders what if.

Part of Johnson's argument is how history's greatest breakthroughs, from Ford's Model T to Darwin's evolution theory, are the climax of multiple eurekas over time. Gutenberg's aha, he'd argue, did not occur in a vacuum. The silversmith had long been grappling with the printing problem, testing ideas in his workshop for years prior to the vineyard visit. Even the wine press was only a few adjustments shy of the printing revolution, the engineering steadily nearing the next big idea.

Across generations we see the adjacent possible. Across a puzzle, we see how one answer can nourish the next. Consider the steam-powered industrial loom of Joseph Jacquard in the early 1800s, an apparatus to spawn the template for Charles Babbage's difference engines, the proto-computers of the 1840s. From loom to calculator to computer: one advance leads to the next, in a single mind or across many.

Suzana Herculano-Houzel, a Brazilian neuroscientist, showed this eureka-chain vividly when confronting a long-standing brain conundrum. As part of her TED talk in 2013, Herculano-Houzel confessed to being curious about the number of neurons found inside the human brain. Everywhere she looked, every coworker she asked, seemed to suggest the grand tally stood at 100 billion, just as I did on this book's preliminary tour, yet nobody could show how that figure had been reached. 'I went digging through the literature,' she recalled, 'trying to find the original reference for that number, and I could never find it. It seems that nobody had ever actually counted the number of neurons in the human brain, or in any other brain for that matter.'

Said another way, the entire field of neuroscience was built on a fuzzy axiom. Nobody knew for sure how many neurons filled the brain. The common tally of 100 billion was a guess, and guesses are fine as hypotheses, but not what you need as a foundation for composing diligent theories.

Rather than hunches, Herculano-Houzel wanted an integer. Yet how to find it? Where would you start in calculating the neural total? This was a genuine test of mental connection. What other field of learning could offer an exact answer? What other eureka could the Brazilian harness to modify the guesstimate? In the end, the solution was cooking.

'It works like this,' as Suzana explained. 'You take a brain, or part of that brain, and you dissolve it in detergent which destroys the cell membranes, but keeps the cell nuclei intact. So you end up with suspension of free nuclei that looks like this . . .' The speaker pulled a phial

INVENTIVE LINKS

'It is by logic that we prove,' said French mathematician Henri Poincaré. 'And it is by intuition that we discover.' Here are some mental connections that went to trigger innovations:

Eiji Nakatsu, a Japanese engineer, is also an avid birdwatcher. Hence the sleek nose of the *Shinkansen* (or bullet train) mimics a kingfisher's streamlined beak.

The warty edges of a humpback's fin inspired US professor Frank Fish (seriously) to design the nodular blades seen on wind turbines.

Professor Graeme Clark held a grass blade within a spiral shell and started imagining. A few years later, in the late 1970s, the first bionic ear emerged from his Melbourne University lab.

Alfred Fielding and Marc Chavannes were keen to make 3D plastic wallpaper by gluing shower curtains together. By accident, the American engineers invented bubble wrap.

The barcode was inspired by Morse code, with US engineer Norman Woodland elongating the dots and dashes into scan-friendly symbols. (Extra fun fact: scanners read the white 'gaps' in each code, not the black stripes.)

Forty years ago, radio astronomer John O'Sullivan and his CSIRO colleagues were seeking to eavesdrop on the dim echoes of black holes. By 1992, the research helped O'Sullivan to fine-tune what we now call wi-fi.

from her pocket, wagging it like a wand at the TED crowd. Inside the tube was a mouse's brain reduced to cloudy soup. 'The beauty of the soup is you can agitate it'—she rocked the phial—'and distribute those nuclei homogenously through the liquid.' Several samples could now be examined through the microscope, tallying the nuclei and thereby calculating the total count of neurons. 'It's simple, it's straightforward, and it's really fast.' And more exact than the long-standing guess of 100 billion ever was.

Thanks to Herculano-Houzel's creative method, bridging two unlikely banks, she could verify the human brain to own an average of 86 billion neurons. Better yet, the soup also yielded a regional census of our brains, with some 16 billion neurons occupying the cerebral cortex alone. 'And if you consider the cerebral cortex is the seat of functions like awareness, and logical and abstract reasoning,' she argued, 'and that 16 billion is the most neurons than any cortex has, then I think this is the simplest explanation for our remarkable cognitive abilities.'

Across species, humans may well own the most neurons—86 billion is a zoological best—but only on the proviso that we know how to use them. From the world's stage to the puzzle page, the brightest minds unthink and relink. Regardless of the problem, the solution is waiting, if only our mind is prepared.

Thinking in harmony

Before work, Cindy liked to solve a crossword. But one morning the usual puzzle in her shoulder bag had been replaced with a sheet of paper. What was going on?

Richard, her English boyfriend, had made a puzzle of his own. Quirky and gentle Richard was always springing small surprises like this. The two twenty-somethings had met in London—the Australian working in events, the boy studying to be a planetary scientist. The couple clicked, their planets aligning as they explored London together. They could chat for hours about everything and nothing. But it was a mutual love of crosswords that lent their meeting a feel of destiny.

Cindy was more at home with quicks—a proficient solver with a wealth of synonyms and a far-ranging vocabulary. Richard, on the other hand, was a cryptic nut. He knew each setters' styles, the standard abbreviations that clues might summon, from hearts (H) to love (O). As a team, their solving powers were multiplied. For that's the SHAZAM factor of crosswording: two brains are better than one. Outsiders assume solving is a solo activity, yet soon we'll visit a few groups who explode that myth, as well as uncover the benefits to your brain of collective solving. But let's return to Cindy and Richard, since crosswords can also lead to lifelong friendship.

Over time, over clues, the romance flourished. They moved to Sydney, and continued to solve crosswords as a mutual hobby. Now and then, just for a cackle, Richard made his own clues for Cindy to solve. Like now as, fifteen minutes before work, Cindy found a strange piece of paper in her bag.

Doubly strange, since most of the clues were missing, while others were breezy by Richard's standards. Like this one:

Writer may whinge despairingly = HEMINGWAY

A lenient anagram—fun but hardly twisted. So what was the catch? The morning turned weirder when a Christmas card arrived at work—in January—from an anonymous sender. Inside the card were more clues, tougher this time.

An hour later, a girlfriend sent Cindy a text. Somehow, in the middle of her chat, her friend mentioned Ovid, the Roman poet. Bingo: OVID was another answer in the crossword.

When Cindy met Richard after work, she begged to know what was happening. By way of explanation, Richard dug in his satchel, fishing out more clues.

Cindy was warming to the game, whatever the game was. The grid was coming together, as they solved clues over wine and ravioli, like these:

Heard sweet rapper? = EMINEM
I sound like an Indian one but noisier? = MINER

Finally two answers remained, but there were no more clues in sight. As the mystery deepened, they drove to a mate's house after dinner. Cindy saw a sci-fi novel in the hall—*Eon* by Greg Bear—which she hated, as Richard knew. Far too galactic, she reckoned—all reincarnation and genetic engineering.

'It's worth a read,' said Richard, handing her the book.

Cindy passed it back, underwhelmed.

'Seriously, take a look,' he said.

Inside was a bookmark with both sides scribbled with code, strings of letters and numbers. Cindy guessed the garble belonged to some sucker hoping to fathom the novel, but then she noticed the pattern:

P63L12W5L4
P104L9W3L5

Page, line, word, letter. Page, line, word, letter. Cindy kept her nerve and calculated the final message to read: LOVE YOU.

Sorry, not final, but penultimate, since I was Richard's accomplice in providing the last piece in this romantic escapade. Cindy, invited to check her email, found my message in the inbox:

Fever seizes ring by Richard initially, ad infinitum (7)

The recipe, she twigged, was a container clue, with ring (O) by Richard initially (R) sit inside FEVER, helping to spell the grid's last entry: FOREVER. By then the boy was on one knee, a piece of bling in his hands. He asked her the day's easiest question apparently, sweetly and un-cryptically, and Cindy said yes.

Room 1, Level 1

Isabelle is 85, a scientist born in New Zealand. Her husband John is only slightly younger, an Aussie engineer and amateur magician. (The man once performed the Chinese rings trick in Melbourne's Savoy Hotel, unlinking and relinking a series of metallic hoops before a rapt audience.) He and Isabelle met back in 1959, in their early 20s, a-la Cindy and Richard—but this time John was the cryptic newbie. 'Isabelle's dad was keen on puzzles in *The Dominion*, I remember, as well as *The New Zealand Listener*. I met Isabelle when I was on a six-month placement in Christchurch and she slowly taught me how to read the clues.'

Isabelle would sit down on weekends with her father, a teapot and crossword between them. 'Dad and I would discuss clues and their solutions and naturally I became interested as well.' Isabelle's eyes light up. 'One clue I recall went something like: "*Chips for one, usually done in oil, and much appreciated.*" The answer was OLD MASTER, after the film *Mr Chips*, and of course the oil paintings of old masters.'

Fittingly, that's what John and Isabelle have become—masters of cryptic language, though don't call them old. In fact, they don't seem old, two Melburnians prompt with a smile and a wry remark, both deeply affectionate towards each other.

Every two weeks, the pair climbs the stairs of Ross House on

SOLVING AS RESOLVING

Deirdre W. and her dad had a major falling out. Umbrage became a summer-long stand-off, and then, while seldom chatty at the best of times, father and daughter fell into a wordless rift lasting many years, long after the first infraction was forgotten.

Salvation arrived in a box, 15 by 15 squares. Through a puzzle, the two had an excuse to make a call, to get back in touch and reignite the conversation. Thanks to a sly reversal, a sneaky definition, the two could whine in harmony, compare notes and share solutions.

'My dad doesn't find it easy to show affection,' wrote Deirdre, 'although I know how strongly it's there. We share a language and an interest, and now we have the reason to spend time together. We can express our love by throwing the page in the other's lap and saying "Have a look at twelve down".'

Flinders Lane, Isabelle's sciatica permitting, armed with the Friday puzzle. With my puzzle, in fact, which is how I came to meet them. First on the page, and then in person while visiting the U3A Cryptic Crossword (Advanced) class one morning.

U3A stands for University of the Third Age. To quote the campus charter, 'The term "University" is used in the original and mediaeval sense of a community of teachers and scholars, united in the pursuit of knowledge.' This communal sense is evident the minute you crest the stairs. I walk into a room of engaged minds and busy pencils. The class has a floating population of two dozen. People come when they can. Today there is a circle of fourteen solvers, a copy of the day's puzzle like a placemat in front of each student. Epiphanies are shared, and thereby deepened.

'Prune!' hollers Felicity, a meteorologist in her late 60s. The room is hers. 'Twenty-one down: *"Shorten jog in gym".*'

'How does it work?' asks Angela, an urban planner in her early 70s. She came to puzzles 'partly as a finite and fun task to enable me to procrastinate from my PhD'.

Felicity unpacks the ruse. 'Shorten is the definition. Another word for jog is run. Put that in PE, which is short for gym . . . '

'Physical education,' adds Joan, 92. She learnt how to solve cryptics when staying on Magnetic Island in 1956.

'The whole thing gives you PRUNE.'

'Prune,' the room murmurs in agreement, elated by the progress, as pencils inscribe the letters, the crossword steadily yielding to the tribal will. As the hour passes, and more clues are tackled, I mentally jog through a checklist of recommendations for all-round brain health. This is the kind that Dementia Australia issued, back in the chapter on memory, where stimuli such as reading, learning, music and puzzle-play were ranked as highly as a healthy diet and regular exercise.

Look at the crossword collective in this light: twice a month they walk upstairs to stretch their brains over 32 clues, give or take, but also to meet with friends, exchange news and share photos of grandchildren. Indeed, socialising is no less a part of the therapy this crew calls a hobby. In 2011, the Rush Alzheimer's Disease Center in Chicago released its findings from a longitudinal study, a health survey conducted over ten years. During that time, some 1138 people with an average age of 79 were canvassed on their lifestyles, and gauged on their cognitive wellbeing.

Points were afforded for each social marker, be that restaurant-going, church services, classes, clubs or even the local bingo. As lead author on the project, Bryan James, explains, 'We were able to look at not just changes in cognition, but changes in social activity. That way we were able to see which preceded the other.'

The results were compelling. According to the data, the greater a subject's social engagement, the stronger their defences against cognitive deterioration. For every one-point increase on the social scorecard, there was a 47 per cent drop in that person's rate of cognitive decline. The more gregarious outliers in the study enjoyed a 70 per cent reduction in the rate of decline.

James concludes, 'Socialising relieves stress, and there's a huge connection between stress and problems with the brain as we get older.' The clue for this is there in our brains. Primates in general, compared to all other orders, own a bigger neocortex. Among the non-humans in that order, the more social members such as baboons and bonobos possess larger cortices. Topping the list, boasting the largest cortex of all, is the human animal. According to James, speaking to *Time* magazine, 'Our brains may be evolved for knowing about 150 people. If you only interact with one or two people, it may not be what we evolved to do.'

So meeting up with friends every few weeks to interact, and swap stories, and decode a cryptic crossword, is a very positive step. Kelvin Edwards, 84, was guiding the group that first day I came, a former teacher in 'real life' and a gifted musician in his own right. Handy as well; the bloke once built a harpsichord from scratch, a shed project he pursued somewhere between his PhD on literacy and developing a love for calligraphy.

At my elbow as I write this book is Kelvin's clue-primer, sealed in plastic, every page presenting a different list of cryptic recipes, from anagrams to charades to 'Additions, Omissions, Etc.' While it was handwritten, Kelvin has rendered each list in a different script: container clues, say, are arrayed in Gothic. Double meanings, Corinthian. And so-called Head Scratchers are full-blown Spencerian.

It's a cryptic book of love, all the dearer for the mentor's death in 2016. The news landed heavily in my inbox. At the memorial service off Grieve Parade (seriously, Kelvin would have loved that), I found myself surrounded by familiar faces. The U3A classroom had migrated to the Chapel of Repose in Altona. Eulogies were marbled with stories of 'Dad's' or 'Poppa's' wordplay, his boundless sense of fun, how the man loved making kites and corny jokes.

Next door in the tearoom, a battered Oxford Dictionary sat among the lamingtons, plus a pre-loved thesaurus, a dog-eared cyclopaedia. The cryptic solvers (Advanced) gravitated towards these sacraments, and remembered.

Two weeks later, they again climbed the stairs of Ross House—John and Isabelle, Joan and Felicity, Robert and Angela, Ian and Cathy, each pilgrim armed with another thorny puzzle to unpick—and they socialised. And they co-solved. In Room 1, Level 1, they kept the flame alive, the memories and epiphanies, the groans and minced oaths, together.

Esprit de core

Other clans assemble in other corners, the magnet of a puzzle exerting its pull. Over the years I've met anaesthetists who animate operations with cryptic grabs: their recipe for staying alert. Professional actors likewise depend on solving clues during rehearsals, the crossword a tonic compared to the distraction of a novel, where a competing narrative stands to blur your focus on the script.

And every Friday a certain software company in Sydney seems deserted as its programmers gather for a makeshift workshop at the café downstairs. 'Back in 2008,' recalls Neo, using his codename in case his boss ever realises how many hours are sacrificed to cryptic lore, 'we had rival solving groups. At lunchtime, there'd be two tables set up for a crossword showdown. Yet we've grown closer over time and just have one group these days.'

Group solving is an act of alchemy—working as a team can elicit the best in everybody, with one person's idle remark levering loose another's idea, which leads to a third's sudden insight. So many minds focused on one grid will ferment a rare blend of competition and cooperation. As a team player you're out to shine as much as support, proving yourself a valued member of the coterie, someone who's both savvy and simpatico.

The scientific term for this is pro-social behaviour. Locked in this dynamic, a weird mojo can descend on any clue. I know this first-hand: facing a stumper you'll be getting nowhere as a solo solver, yet the minute you share the clue with a friend—vocalise it, theorise it—the subterfuge fractures and the light spills in.

Parallels between solving and coding are not lost on Neo. 'We see some aspects of our programming culture appearing in our crossword group. We have a "driver" who reads the clues and wields the pen. There's a lot of time spent by individuals thinking about the clues and taking it apart themselves, suggesting ideas and seeing what people

TWO'S COMPANY—U3A'S A CLASS

The University of the Third Age (aka U3A) began life in Toulouse back in 1973, ensuring elder minds didn't get rusty in retirement. Since then the movement has blossomed across some forty nations.

Melbourne was home to the first Australian campus in 1984, with each state swiftly following suit. At last count, enrolments hovered at around 85,000 students coast to coast, in courses including languages, computing, philosophy, current affairs, yoga, bridge and the ever-popular wine appreciation. To learn more about learning, or where your nearest U3A campus can be found, visit <www.u3aonline.org.au/find-a-u3a?combine=Australia>.

latch on to. So there is a similarity there in that group work can help a bit, but individuals ultimately solve the problems.'

Or do they? That's the ongoing debate in some pockets of psychology. Journalist James Surowiecki, in his 2004 book *The Wisdom of Crowds*, argues a crowd holds 'a nearly complete picture of the world in its collective brain'. But the more diverse the crowd the greater the chances of success. When a team comprises like experts—solely IT programmers, say—the group can be prone to exploiting a single vein of knowledge. With a wider sampling of intelligent people, like the Ross House brigade, or the complementary strengths of Cindy and Richard, there's greater potential for exploration.

Rather than choose puzzles to underscore his point, Surowiecki opted for a nuclear submarine. In 1968, the USS *Scorpion* vanished in the Atlantic between Spain and Rhode Island. Locating the vessel felt as improbable as winning the lottery until John Craven, a scientist attached to the US Navy, assembled a group of thinkers—from oceanographers to mathematicians—and set them a real-life puzzle. If you had to draw an X in the sea, the likely place to find the sub, then where would it be?

Importantly, all the elements of an effective group dynamic were in place:

Diversity—no member of the group shared the same string of letters after their name, and therefore carried a healthy store of 'private information'.

Decentralisation—no wild-eyed admiral ruled the meeting with that top-down tyranny of some workplaces we might know.

Independence—everyone's thoughts mattered as much as the next sub-hunter's.

Aggregation—some means existed for everyone's smart guess to be melded into a smarter one.

The submarine hunt ran more in line with a guessing game than a brainstorm seeking a prescribed answer.

Neo calls it hypothesis-forming, a skill integral to programming and crosswording. Working in isolation, in the office or the grid, you need to process the invisible algebra alone—test option A, only to dismiss A, and move on to option B, or J, or Q, whichever might satisfy the equation. This is healthy exercise for the brain, but add a colleague, a lover, a dozen classmates, and the puzzle sparks an open laboratory of tested speculations, trialled and trashed in record time.

It sounds ruthless, but I saw no such thing in Room 1, Level 1—and can't imagine knives being hurled in the café of a certain IT giant. To the contrary, every solver I quizzed for this book talked of love and enjoyment when describing the practice of puzzling.

And let's not forget Christine Hooker's revelations, back in 2010. Hooker was the assistant professor of psychology at Harvard, the researcher to link puzzle-solving with rapprochement among disgruntled couples. If we use the prefrontal cortex more often—whether that's to wrestle sudokus or moderate anger—we gain a greater ability to overcome ill feelings, and preserve an *esprit de corps*.

The evidence is in, both the anecdotal and academic: crosswords can bring people closer together, whether that entails falling in love or keeping the brain limber into your third age. They can inspire wedding proposals or noontide cabals. They can expedite forgiveness or see two groups coalesce.

But wait there's more: even if you solve a crossword in isolation, away from the crowd, set apart from your partner, the same activity will exercise your *latent carpal rotor reflex*, which regular bouts of brain-bending will tell you is an anagram of *lateral prefrontal cortex*, the very chamber that accommodates good relations.

As for that submarine, I won't leave you in limbo. Craven combined his team's individual guesses into one collective estimate. In the end, while no member of the group pinpointed the stricken vessel, the derived X was only 200 metres from where the actual wreck was eventually found—a mere 200 metres in an open sea of 106,460,000 square metres. That's some guesswork.

So no matter the puzzle—a shipwreck, a sequence of matches, a memory-bender, a cryptic clue—enigmas help us think. And keep thinking.

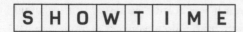

Juggling is good for both reflex and cortex, according to a study conducted by a team at the University of Oxford in 2009. While honing the circus skill has some pretty obvious benefits—improved peripheral vision and general coordination to name two—the researchers also claimed it grows your brain.

Twenty-four subjects, none of whom could juggle, were split into two groups. Over six weeks, one group took a crash course in juggling, with weekly lessons to supplement their own daily half-hour practice sessions. The other group, acting as the control, learnt zilch, as oblivious of juggling as when they first volunteered.

To open and close the research, each participant was given an fMRI scan: the clinical equivalent of before and after photos. The images allowed Dr Heidi Johansen-Berg, the study's lead, to gauge whether any brain-changes had occurred during the interim.

Among the trainee jugglers, the news was encouraging. As Johansen-Berg summarised, '[Our study suggests] that in healthy adults, learning a new skill over a relatively short period of six weeks is changing the brain; it's changing the size of brain areas involved in the task, and it's changing the wiring between different brain areas.'

To be specific, each juggler's brain displayed increased density in the myelin sheath, the pale cellular matter that insulates our axons, while the juggling muggle—the non-learner—displayed the same brain as before.

The media cheered. Juggling is beneficial, read every spin-off article. Though Johansen-Berg was quick to temper the hype: 'This doesn't mean that everyone should go out and start juggling to improve their brains. We chose juggling purely as a complex new skill for people to learn.'

Replace juggling for crossword solving, and the repercussions follow. While jumbling letters and double-meaning won't improve your chances of catching your Vegemite toast before it hits the lino, the new-found skill is bound to boost your mental agility, your semantic memory, your problem-solving and every other dimension that Part One has touched on.

Like the juggling study, the data surrounding the act of solving isn't foolproof but it is optimistic, every sign suggesting the custom is nourishing the mind. And unlike juggling, ten times the research has been held in puzzle-play, with each paper confirming that the solver's brain is a boosted brain, as nimble as an acrobat.

The only thing lacking now is a circus ring where you can put your skills to the test. For all the promises of Part One, the real show hasn't started. To be a lion tamer, you need to find a chair and tame a lion. That's where Part Two does the trick, where talk of brain health plays second fiddle to hands-on letter juggling.

I've already tossed a few curveballs your way, a few sidebar puzzles by way of rehearsal, giving your brain a sense of solving solo in the spotlight. So far, in earlier chapters, I've served up pun-clues and alphagrams, memory games and celebrity cocktails: how many answers did you catch?

Not that it matters—you're a juggler in training. Clumsiness is natural. Besides, if this book was a circus manual, then you'd need some props. Rubber chickens to lob. Skittles and balls. Everything till now has been a barker's cry, a drum-roll to lure you into the tent, making the call for practice overdue.

I could be dogmatic, of course. I could say:

Step one: Bundle two socks into a ball.
Step two: Hold the ball in one hand, standing over a bed or table, and toss the bundle upwards.
Step three: Catch the ball in your hand.
Step four: Repeat.

And so on. Throw, catch, throw, repeat. As soon as the neurons have started firing in sync, we could graduate to lobbing two bundles. Next step: chainsaws.

But this language would be wasted without the props on hand. After Part One, we all know puzzling is good for the brain, so what say we puzzle? Let's roll up, roll up, and enter Part Two, all the better to furnish your big top.

Johansen-Berg, the juggling researcher, concluded her findings with a familiar tune: 'There is a "use it or lose it" school of thought, in which any way of keeping the brain working is a good thing, such as going for a walk or doing a crossword.'

That's our cue, folks. It's showtime.

THE

HOW-TO

Unlocking a cryptic crossword

Getting your brain puzzle-fit

Despite everything you hear, or whatever you presume, cryptic crosswords aren't that hard. Let me say that again: cryptic crosswords aren't that hard. With one big if: *if you know how to read the clues*.

The moment you attune to the language, the eurekas flow. Veteran solvers know that already. Each clue has rules to obey. To an outsider, this may seem unlikely, given the puzzles read like gibberish, but there's a hidden grammar awaiting your mind.

Chess is a good parallel. As a kid, glancing at a chessboard from a distance, I panicked. The game had no apparent logic. Different pieces had different mannerisms, from sliding castles to jumping horses. A pawn might move one square, or two, or cut a diagonal path if it wished to kill a bishop. Every contest seemed a genteel sort of chaos.

That changed the moment I grasped chess's rules. As soon as I gleaned the principles—learnt where the pieces stand and how they travel—the chaos dissipated.

Of course, learning the rules of chess is not the same as mastering the game, which might take a lifetime. But the argument still holds: grasp the ABCs of KQB, and you can savour chess from the inside, enjoying the battle rather than battling to understand.

It's not far to jump from a chessboard to a cryptic crossword. To fathom the clues, you need to read the instructions, which you'll meet on the pages to come.

Or maybe you know the basics already and wish to improve your solving insights. Either way, the tools await you in Part Two.

That's why I've split this section into four, five if we count this preamble. Coming up is a choice of tutorials, arranged according to your solving prowess. Novices should start at the lowest level, getting familiar with the basic clue formulas, before attempting the more advanced workout, where hardcore solvers are invited to begin. Or then again, even if you're a dab hand already, you may well enjoy seeing the start-up stuff, if not to refresh your memory, then to measure the progress you've made since coming to the puzzle page.

The tutorials are as follows:

Body building is a brisk rundown of how a clue is made, a blueprint recommended for every reader. This section will show you how to scan a cryptic clue, and how to break it down. Learners will need to know this discipline, while experts will benefit from seeing the familiar principles revisited. After that comes your workout dilemma—the *Neuro-cardio* gentle start-up or the *Guru yoga* high-intensity training? Both courses teem with chances to stretch your wits and boost your brainpower for the wrestles to follow.

Neuro-cardio is a crash course for rookies, a chance to meet the most common recipes from anagrams to deletions. No stopwatch, no deadline—the circuit is there for you to get familiar with each mode of cryptic language, from reversals to charades, grasping the elements of each clue type, and alerting your senses to the regular traps.

Guru yoga, on the other hand, is more of a stretch. Made for cryptic insiders, this level tests your reflexes across a rarer range of clues, dipping into spoonerisms, entangling with puns and overhauling rebuses. By going deeper into the craft of crosswords, this session will help you glean the setter's mindset, seeing all the moves and poses that go behind the deceits.

Your sessions await, custom-made for the tyro or the pro. And when you've sweated through one or both, then I can recommend Part Two's last hurrah—the *Booster pack*, comprising the top ten tips for solving success. Treat this final checklist as a touchstone. If need be, fit the pack into your pocket to keep brain-fit for the real stuff coming. Let's crack on.

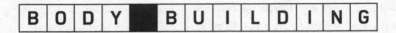

BODY BUILDING

How cryptic clues work

The best way to see how cryptic clues work is to look at how they don't work. Rather than start with the curly stuff, getting too messy with manipulations, let's focus on the so-called quick crossword. As you know, simple clues give you the answer's definition and nothing more. Like so:

Bug (6)

No mess, no fuss, but what's the answer?

INSECT obviously fits, yet so does HORNET and CICADA. Which guess is best?

That's the catch: quick clues aren't really that quick. Unless a clue is bleeding obvious—like *Christmas month* (8)—then you can't guarantee which synonym will do the trick. Often the clue is too bare, giving you too little traction to test one hunch over another.

In fact, the more you contemplate *bug*, the longer your list grows. What about LOCUST or SPIDER? SCARAB or WEEVIL?

Or maybe it's *bug* as in virus—like GRIPPE or AMOEBA, STRAIN or DENGUE.

Or possibly *bug* the verb, a synonym of annoy, which summons such possibilities as BOTHER or HASSLE, HARASS or BADGER, RANKLE or PESTER.

You get the gist. There's nothing quick about a quick crossword.

Even when a letter arrives, the risks remain. Say E is confirmed as the final letter of your mystery *bug*, courtesy of a cross-running answer, making this pattern on paper:

_ _ _ _ _ E

Finally, a chance to pin the bug down, but even now ample suspects still remain. Words like NEEDLE or NETTLE surface, or even NIGGLE. As candidates go, you can't blank BEETLE or RUFFLE, PLAGUE or TSETSE. One stab feels as good as the next.

Compare that muddle to a cryptic crossword. Instead of a prosaic definition, a cryptic clue offers two chances of snaring the one answer—a straight path and a twisty path that both end up at the same destination. Keeping things buggy, consider this specimen:

Squashed nicest bug (6)

Remember, don't fall for the story. Newbies will picture some lovely butterfly splattered by a shoe, or a ladybird mushed beneath a tyre, but that is the clue's deception. Viewing any clue as a story is diverting your brain from the challenge of solving.

So don't be a sucker. Go below the surface. To crack a cryptic, you must abandon the literal. Be suspicious. Unpeel the picture offered and switch your brain to a lateral setting. Do it right, and you get *inside* the clue.

Ninety-nine per cent of cryptic clues have two parts. (Let's not worry about the exceptions for now.) Without fail, those two parts are the definition and the wordplay. One part will *define* the answer—just like a quick crossword—and the other will *play with* the answer. Like the two parts in the brain, one hemisphere will be logical (the definition), and the other creative.

Merge them and you have a cryptic clue—a marriage of the conventional and the playful, where both parts work together to pinpoint the answer.

So long as you can work out which part is which. Let's return to that bug situation:

Squashed nicest bug (6)

Wangling the wording one small degree, you get this:

Squashed nicest / bug (6)

As trivial as that slash might seem, it's vital. In brain terms, it's the fissure that separates the two hemispheres, isolates the two modes of thinking. Notice the parts aren't the same in length? That asymmetry is common in cryptic clues and the reason I've been avoiding the word halves.

As a solver, the virtual surgeon on the page, you must discern where to cut. Slice the right gap and the clue will open up. A neat line, at the right point, will separate the definition from the wordplay, or vice versa, exposing the two pathways to the single answer.

Here the slash exposes the definition (*bug*) at the clue's end, which means the clue's remainder is the riddle element—the wordplay aiming at a six-letter word set to satisfy the definition. Feel free to crack either part, since the answer for both is the same.

Or solve one part, and check that answer against the other part, because cryptic clues are handy that way, allowing you to confirm your hunch, unlike those nasty quick crosswords, which can bug the brain with nothing but a dictionary grab, giving you no further means of verifying your response.

In case you haven't guessed, the wordplay recipe found in our sample clue is the anagram. *Squash* NICEST, as the wordplay is telling us, and you can make a new word meaning bug. Go ahead.

Soon those six letters in NICEST will metamorphose into INSECT, the very first theory we floated when facing the quick version—but this time you know it's right, thanks to the definition sitting next door. There's no need to recite all those other suspects, the beetles and rankles on your list, since the cryptic clue comes with its own confirmation. How nice is that?

Anagrams, I should add, are just one style of wordplay you'll meet on the cryptic page. Indeed, that opening clue in the Florey trial belonged to the anagram family, namely:

Organised relay in good time (5)

The answer is EARLY, as my brain spotted in less than two seconds. How long did your brain take, reorganising the letters of RELAY to make good time?

Coming up in this first section are seven more recipe types, including anagrams, plus more eccentric variations. But before we sample other styles, here's one more clue with an insect flavour:

Insect plague I wager (6)

Again, you need to play surgeon, testing where to plant the scalpel. And again, the anagram formula is in action.

As an experiment, perhaps try a few different cuts? You end up with these choices:

Insect / plague I wager
Insect plague / I wager
Insect plague I / wager

Which part is most likely to provide an anagram of the answer? And which part seems to answer best as a definition?

Those questions lie central to the cryptic mindset. Sense how a clue is made, which word is playing what role, and you're almost touching the solution. The more you dismantle the language, the sooner you'll identify the seam that holds the parts together—the definition and the wordplay.

Or vice versa: the wordplay and the definition. Don't forget those two parts can appear in either order. In our first example, the wordplay was first, where NICEST needed squashing. And here, in this last teaser, the definition opens the clue:

Insect plague I wager (6)

Insect or *insect plague*? You'd plausibly meet both in a dictionary, but in this case plague has a different role to fulfil. Here the word's a signpost (as crossword setters call it), otherwise termed an anagram indicator, or compressed into anagrind, just like *squashed* in the first example.

So you've made it this far. What next? You obey the clue and, bearing in mind the answer is six letters long, you plague the six nearby letters *I wager*.

But wait, you ask. Why not plague I-N-S-E-C-T to spell the solution? That also has six letters. A fair point, though that reading would mean the answer's definition would be the remaining *I wager*. Not impossible, but hardly likely.

Therefore it's smarter to wrangle I-W-A-G-E-R, aiming for *insect* as the definition. Give it a whirl, literally. See what insect emerges.

Have you found it? As a bonus hint, consider a hairy listener. Too cryptic? Okay then, your solution starts with E this time. Does that help? Bug-wise, the answer's biological order is *Dermaptera*, though most of us know this pincered pest as an EARWIG.

And there you have it—a brisk run-through of The Cryptic Rule of Two, the definition and the wordplay (or vice versa). To become a cryptic master, you must move away from the literal-think of simple clues, as well as simple stories, and heed the wording's deeper purpose. Train your brain to think that way, and I guarantee the bug will bite.

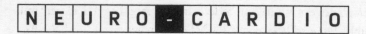

A cryptic crash course

This chapter is a tour of the mental gymnasium, a breezy intro to the various pieces of cryptic equipment on the ground floor. You've already met anagrams, the most common of the brain-benders. Soon we'll grapple with that formula at greater length—just to etch a neural pathway for all those hours of future puzzle-play—and then continue the circuit, testing our wits on seven other exercises, from charades to homophones.

Once you get a grip on all eight categories, you can either try your luck with the puzzles in Part Three straightaway, or, alternatively, for a full-body workout, you can graduate to 'Guru yoga', the advanced solving session.

Care to flex before we start? Grab a glass of water, a sweat towel, a quick banana? Your grey matter is set to stretch to snapping point—in a good way, of course. I'm only trying to train your cortex for the main event to come. Take a deep breath and let the brain-stretching begin.

Anagrams

I love how SNAKE holds SNEAK, or NOSTALGIA is a blend of LOST AGAIN, or GREASEPAINT hides in PAGEANTRIES. This is the simple reward of anagrams, where so many words can hide their alter ego, like TREADMILL whispering I MELT LARD, or FAD DIET confessing DIED FAT!

I totally dig how LANDSCAPING is made up of SCAN, PLAN and DIG—the holy trinity of rejuvenating a garden. Or how FIDGET SPINNER—the momentary madness of 2017—conceals its customary location: FINGERTIP'S END.

Though not every anagram reflects its source. RESCUED may well nestle in SECURED, just as PARENTAL can generate PATERNAL, but linking ASTRONAUT to ROAST TUNA seems a giant leap, and let's not touch ADULTERY and TRUE LADY.

Still, the game is addictive, and underpins this popular formula. We've already met a few bugs in this vein, from the NICEST INSECT to an EARWIG, I WAGER. And if you recall, both example clues included a signpost that told you to mix—the anagram indicator.

You see the same thing in this clue from Orlando, a long-time setter for *The Guardian*:

Shopkeeper bursting into tears (9)

Previously, you might have been fooled by this clue. Fed a diet of quick crosswords and paperback novels, you may have fallen for the narrative. *Awww, the poor shopkeeper—is he alright? Why's he weeping? Did his cat die?*

Not now. Now your brain is adapting to a new way of thinking. Now you sift the language for signs of the lurking anagram. Orlando's clue has two possible signposts—*bursting* and *tears*. (And don't think the salty sort of tears, but rips and scratches. Reject the story and rethink the potential of each and every word.) So then, which sign do you obey?

Asked another way, which indicator sits adjacent to the likely batch of nine letters, the raw materials to build the solution? *Shopkeeper* has ten letters, so we can rule that word out as fodder (crossword-speak for the letters needed to make the anagram, the pieces that deliver the whole). If *tears* was the signpost, then there's no adjacent fodder to jumble that owns the right amount of letters.

Hence the spotlight lingers on the phrase *into tears*, a neat nine letters. Could they be our fodder?

If so, then they hide a nine-letter word. Better still, if our theory is sound, that word means shopkeeper, the only part of the clue yet to be assigned a role.

Those earlier bug clues showed that no word is wasted in a cryptic clue, not a scrap, not a syllable. Every word has a secret mission to fulfil. Your job as solver is working out what those roles are.

Have you found that missing shopkeeper? Mixing nine letters in the brain is probably about three letters too many for most mortals. It can be extra difficult when distracted, so fetch some paper and a pen. Jot down those nine letters: INTOTEARS.

Notice I said nine letters, not two words. Because INTOTEARS may as well be TIRONSTEA, or NESTITORA. Why abide by their original order? The phrase is not a phrase anymore, but an overlong Scrabble rack, the clue telling you to burst the batch into something new—a shopkeeper.

SIENATROT. TSOAIRNTE. AEINORSTT . . .

Another approach many solvers try is the wheel method, spinning the fodder into a loose array, the easier to see the letters' potential:

$$I \quad R \quad T$$
$$A \quad S \quad T \quad N$$
$$O \quad E$$

Does that help?

Unless the answer is a brand, or notable retailer's surname, the nine-letter shopkeeper is likely to be a job ending in IST, such as pharmacist or florist. Or maybe ER, like grocer or bookdealer.

We call this cluster theory. It's handy in the anagram game. You look at the meaning of the mystery word—in this case shopkeeper—and surmise what shape the solution will take. If the definition is pasta, then try combinations ending in I or A. If sport is mentioned, don't ignore BALL or ING. Tempos often end in O, just as beliefs finish with ISM, and dinosaurs, AURUS. Not always, but these patterns recur. Books and films, by the same token, often open with THE, while a slew of synthetics kick off with POLY or end in ENE. It's hardly the stuff of a Nobel Prize, but testing out clusters can be a great shortcut in finding your answer.

And what is our answer? It's time to unmask Orlando's shopkeeper. After your anagram practice, should you need more paper, you may need to visit your local STATIONER.

Now let's push the envelope further to see how you cope with eight more anagram clues from various sources, including a few of my own.

S I G N P O S T S ▮ ▯ ▯ ▯ ▮ ▯ ▯ ▯ ▮

ANAGRAM (a sampling)

abroad	ground	renegade
amiss	hammer	rent
anyhow	Harrow	rogue
awfully	impromptu	sabotage
bubbly	in a state	sack
bung	in error	salad
burst	invalid	Scrabble
byzantine	jars	shift
comic	junk	shiver/ing
complex	knit	shot
compound	knot	sorry
correct	liberal	splurge
corrupt	marshal	spray
crude	misbehaving	stray
derelict	mobile	structure
deviant	mongrel	stuff
disorder	motion	stunning
distress	on the loose	supply (in a supple way!)
do	otherwise	suspect
doctor	out to lunch	swimming
eccentric	plastic	tangled
failing	position	tattoo
flaky	potty	trip
fluid	pound	vagrant
foreign	prepare	WAGs
founder	pulp	waves
fragments	rash	wear/ing
fraudulent	recollected	wind
Gaga	recreation	windy
go off	Reformation	wrought

As all eight entail the anagram recipe, look for the likely signposts (any words suggesting change or disarray), plus the likely fodder, which must sit immediately to the left or right of the signpost.

To boost your anagram cracking, take time to browse the box above for common signposts, noting how some (like doctor or plastic) are slyly camouflaged.

Oh wait, one more thing before we meet the examples. Now and then, a standard anagram clue is made more advanced by adding a conjunction, typically 'and' or 'with'. It's nothing to worry about—just an extra hurdle to clear. One example comes from *Times* puzzle 10,977:

Mirror for one, old and a bit cracked (7)

It's a beautiful subterfuge, the clue's surface as polished as a factory-new mirror. But if that mirror is *old and a bit cracked*, then you're wise to ignore the linking word of *and*, and so identify the seven-letter anagram fodder as OLDABIT. Equally, you'd be smart to unthink shiny surfaces and antique looking-glasses, despite the seductive story, and consider *mirror* in another setting. Look more deeply. Think more widely. Consider *for one*—the phrase—as a further clue, the wording inviting you to treat mirror as a category example, being one among others of its kind. Sure enough, *Mirror* with a capital M, say, is a very different object. Not cracked but racked, lodged on Fleet Street's newsstands. Sure enough, the moment you crack OLDABIT—skipping the clue's conjunction—you get TABLOID.

E	X	A	M	P	L	E	S							

Anagram

1. *Rocky terrain footwear* (7) [Gila]
2. *Bird place in resort* (7) [DA]
3. *Showed doctor he's rude* (7) [Arachne]
4. *Urged on wild bear* (7) [Imogen]
5. *Stewed over rap song idea* (8) [DA]
6. *Halt cannon shot, showing composure* (10) [*Times* 10,786]
7. *Unwind with large one in pub* (8,4) [Toro]
8. *Fried dish cook made with a pan* (8) [*Times* 10,348]

[Note—the asterisk is used beside solutions to signal the anagram mode.
The information in square brackets after each clue reveals the setter/source.]

ANSWERS 1. TRAINER*, 2. PELICAN*, 3. USHERED*, 4. UNDERGO*, 5. AGONISED*, 6. NONCHALANT*, 7. WATERINGHOLE*, 8. EMPANADA*

The final clue in the eight Anagram examples likewise relies on a conjunction. Just use the letter count to isolate the right fodder, and you'll shuffle with minimal kerfuffle.

Double definitions

A bug can be a cockroach or a listening device. The same word can translate as a germ or a verb, a computer glitch or a Volkswagen model.

Double-definition clues exploit that polysemy, the fancy term for many meanings. English is notorious for polysemy, with so many entries in the dictionary owning multiple senses.

Tears can be eye dribble or holes in your jeans. Pen is a female swan, a sheepfold, a prison or something a stationer sells. Probing deeper, you'll discover gig can mean a performance, a one-horse carriage, a racing boat, a fishing spear, a stickybeak or a data-storage unit.

You get the drift? (And by drift I mean the meaning, not the current's tug, or the car's deviation, or the snowpile . . .)

With more layers than a henhouse, English is custom-made for double-definition clues, a formula cinching two quick clues into one cryptic duet. Here's one twosome:

Clever sting! (5)

This clue is care of Moley, an occasional setter with *The Guardian*. His exclamation mark seeks to dramatise the clue's story and should be ignored, like a lot of punctuation in cryptic clues. (I'll talk some more about punctuation in the chapter 'Guru yoga', with special attention paid to the curly question mark, and what it might suggest. But for now, let's focus on Moley's two words.)

That's right—just two words. Brevity is a common feature of the double-definition formula. If a compiler is clever, she only needs to find the right two words where both selections denote the same solution.

Moley did just that, finding *clever* and *sting* to coin a false head-line. (The exclamation mark seeks to sustain that newsflash veneer.) But really, all the clue is saying is: what one word means both *clever* and *sting*?

If the clue was a quick, you'd only get one of these two:

Clever (5)
Sting (5)

Neither of which will lead to a quick solution, since clever could denote WITTY, SMART, SHARP, CANNY or ADEPT, while sting may mean SCALD, PRICK, SMART, CHILL or PRANK.

Holy moly, did you notice something there? One word is on both lists: SMART is synonym to both *clever* and *sting*.

Compare that certainty to the freefall anxiety of a quick clue, where a single word points to several possibilities. Cryptic clues give you a double helping, allowing you to eliminate such doubts. Quick smart—put SMART in your grid. With ink.

Of course, where beginners need to exercise care is when nuance blurs the picture. A far more devious example of this clue style comes from Screw, also a *Guardian* setter:

In on (9)

Again the minimal length betrays the double-definition recipe. (This is useful to remember as you scan a bed of clues, wondering which recipes lie where, and which ones to unpick first.) And again, the clue's brief length should tell you what you're chasing—a word meaning both *in* and *on*.

Yet both words boast whole pages in the dictionary, so a solver must lean on their *Sprachgeful* (that German word from the 'Vocabulary' chapter, namely a feeling for language). What nine-letter word has both *on* and *in* as synonyms?

To ease your pain, the answer is HAPPENING: slang for fashionable (*in*), and a shorthand way of saying *on*—that is, being performed, or going ahead.

But don't assume that every double-definition clue has only two words. As you'll see, some can run to six or seven words. While this can make the formula harder to detect, the yin-yang principle is the same—two definitions coupling to denote one solution.

One more thing you're bound to notice when tackling double definitions is the absence of a signpost. This makes sense: unlike the anagram mode, there's no scrambling required. By dodging this obligation, the double-definition clue will be leaner than most.

So then, are you game? And by game I mean plucky, not a partridge or polo or a profession . . . Just remember, treat each part as a quick clue, and you should then make an:

Excellent guess (6) = DIVINE

Time for the twins.

E	X	A	M	P	L	E	S								

Double definition

1. *Not in shape* (6) [*Times* 10,987]
2. *Resist money* (4) [Arachne]
3. *Was sulky a basic form of transport?* (5) [Anax]
4. *Sweet stall* (5) [Mudd]
5. *Abridge legal document* (8) [Hectence]
6. *Less sensitive figure* (6) [DA]
7. *Escape death in operation* (4) [Citrus]
8. *Preparing to twerk after rest* (8,2,3,4) [Donk]

ANSWERS: 1. SQUARE, 2. BUCK, 3. MOPED, 4. FUDGE, 5. CONTRACT, 6. NUMBER, 7. LIVE, 8. BRINGING UP THE REAR

Charades

Like double-definition clues, the cryptic charade also lacks a signpost. The reason is simple: just as anagrams swirl and stir, the charade is more about subdivision, breaking answers into smaller units.

If you've ever played charades, you know the drill. With no speaking allowed, the old parlour game relies on gestures to signal a phrase or movie. Take *Charlotte's Web*, for example. The common tactic is to break the name into chunks, turning CHARLOTTES into CHAR+LOTTES, and then acting out the pieces.

'First syllable,' says your guessing team. 'Sounds like . . . sounds like car? Second syllable . . . many? Plenty? Heaps? Oodles . . . ?'

This fracturing routine is also maintained in a cryptic setting. MAINTAIN, say, can be sliced into MAIN, TA and IN. APPROACH breaks into APP and ROACH. Even ANAGRAM resembles a line of farm animals with A NAG beside a RAM.

In case that feels a lot like mixing, note that the charade is more about respacing than recycling. In scientific terms, charades splits ATOM into A TOM, while the anagram mode prefers MOAT. Instead of smashing PARTICLES into CLIP RATES, as anagram clues will do, the charade formula prefers P plus ARTICLES.

For the record, a charade answer can be short (CON+DO) or long (FORT+HERE+CORD). It could be a name (JUST+IN+TIMBER+LAKE), or even divide a compound like SIGNPOST into two fresh meanings of SIGN and POST.

Charades can also be difficult, perhaps the hardest of the introductory recipes. So don't fret if they don't unravel easily; it takes a little practice to detect a charade in the wild, and a lot more time to master them.

To see how these specimens read, let's examine (EX+A+MINE) a charade clue from one of my favourite compilers:

Officer swindles board (9)

The clue hails from the late Henry Hook, a champion compiler from New Jersey who died too young in 2015, aged only 60. 'I got into the [crossword] business to torment people,' he once told the *New Yorker* magazine. Good as his word, Hook could turn an unsuspecting brain into knots.

Perusing Henry's clue, how do you break down the elements? *Swindles* in another setting might serve as an anagram indicator, but that theory has to be abandoned for want of nine adjacent letters to serve as fodder.

With such a short clue, you might suspect a double definition. But your answer would need to be a synonym of *officer swindles* or *swindles board*, and neither adds up. (Can you see the reasoning behind that?

If a double definition is in play, then two of Henry Hook's three words needed to be paired into a single unit. Yet both pairings seem unlikely—*officer swindles* or *swindles board*—so we need to unlock this clue with a different key.)

With your brain humming, you consider the charade recipe, the idea boosted by the lack of obvious signpost. To test the waters you ponder synonyms. That's the secret to cracking charades. Shrewd solvers will consult their mental thesaurus to see what other words can substitute for any in the clue. In Hook's clue, there are three words. Try subbing them, testing out synonyms, with the emphasis on shorter replacements. By shorter I mean six letters or less, since your nine-letter answer will comprise two words.

Officer could be a major, a cop, a dean. *Swindles* could be cons or cheats, dupes or tricks. *Board* suggests plank or table, panel or embark . . .

Your best bet of that list is con (or cons), a fragment common to umpteen English words. Do you know an officer starting with CONS? Or a table ending with CONS?

Officer swindles board (9)

In rental jargon, full board means both accommodation and meals. Board is a quaint synonym for table, where those all-inclusive meals are served. Now add TABLE to CONS, or vice versa, and Hook's undercover officer will flash his badge.

Charade clues demand a good vocab, plus the mental agility to see which synonyms click. Just to keep you guessing, the occasional charade will give you the actual fragment, rather than a synonym, such as:

Can adolescent make mess? (7) = CAN+TEEN

And if that's not sly enough, a charade clue might also enlist a single letter among the pieces, or a cluster of letters that don't necessarily spell a word. WORDS, for one, might be charaded this way:

Terms for women or dames outside = W+OR+DS

Spelt in full, that's W (from *women*, the letter on toilet doors) plus OR plus DS (the *outside* letters of *dames*).

Fear not. You won't be meeting such charades in the short term, but the time seemed right to show you how compact some sequences can be, relying on whole words and fragmentary letters to build the answer.

Sneaky right? See how you MAN+AGE—or COP+E—with these.

E	X	A	M	P	L	E	S								

Charade

1. *Posed wearing glossy fabric* (5) [Columba]
2. *UK actress Kate takes prize with permission* (7) [DA]
3. *UK model Naomi affected inventor* (8) [DA]
4. *Wild sheep breathe heavily* (7) [Emily Cox & Henry Rathvon]
5. *Confused by commercial break* (6) [Portia]
6. *Old Greek building standard formerly in operation* (9) [Henry Hook]
7. *Old Greek philosopher concerned with group of soldiers* (7) [Orlando]
8. *Old friend showing lack of resolution* (9) [Phi]

ANSWERS: 1. SAT+IN, **2.** WINS+LET, **3.** CAMP+BELL, **4.** RAM+PANT, **5.** AD+RIFT, **6.** PAR+THEN+ON, **7.** PLATO+ON, **8.** STALE+MATE

Homophones

Q: Did you hear the one about the homophone recipe?
A: Know. Eye knead yore guy-dunce.

Above is a glimpse of the next mind-trip. Or maybe sound-bite is a better label, since the homophone clue dwells in the audio realm. In welcome news for novices, the recipe demands a signpost, which is often easy to detect. Top of the list are *say* and *hear*, but any word or phrase denoting sound is, well, sound. Check out the box on page 113 for other possible indicators.

The 'reel' trick with homophones is the two-step strategy you need to adopt. To break that down, you must:

(1) Identify the synonym being suggested.
(2) Say that synonym aloud to 'hear' the answer.

S I G N P O S T S

HOMOPHONE (a sampling)

acoustic	noisy	readout
articulate	on tape	registered
by ear	on the phone	related
called	oral	report
catch	oration	reporter's
commentator's	outspoken	so-called
declared/declaration	parrot	talking
of	phoned	tape/d
dictator's	pick up	tell/ing
eavesdrop	picked up	teller's
expressed	pickup	*The Conversation*
in conversation	podcast	*The Voice*
in reception	pronounced	under discussion
in/voice	quoted	verbal
narrator's	read out	vocal

It 'mite' be wiser to show you one in action. Below is a clue by a British setter called Mudd, whose real name is John Halpern, a modern dynamo of cryptic brilliance. Across the mastheads he's known as Paul (*The Guardian*), Punk (*The Independent*), Mudd (*Financial Times*), plus he's a prolific setter for *The Times,* a puzzle whose setters remain uncredited on the page. See how you 'fair' with this offering:

Sound Indian location for shop (4)

Said another way, '*Sound out a place in India to hear a type of shop*'. Unpacked like that, the cryptic clue becomes simpler, since only one obvious candidate emerges. It can't be coal-cutter (Kolkatta) or Pune (pooh-neigh), so it must be Delhi. Utter the city's name aloud and you have the shop: DELI.

The clue is more lenient than others, as it has the audio-signpost right before the denoted word, telling you which word—or synonym—to voice. Homophones get harder if the indicator occupies the clue's middle, such as a recast of Mudd's clue:

Indian location's sound shop (4)

Ordered that way, you need to figure out what needs sounding, the word produced by the left or right side of the indicator. Should a solver wish to decipher this redrafted version, the thinking would follow along these lines:

(1) The possessive apostrophe is saying the sound belongs to the location, not the shop.
(2) The answer has four letters, so Delhi spoken aloud becomes DELI.

Whenever dilemmas occur, answer length is often a handy toehold. Here in Mudd's rejigged clue, if the answer has only four letters, then the synonym (here, the Indian location) must likewise be short. It stands to reason that when single words are involved, the word you say is likely to have approximately the same number of letters, with several of those letters being shared.

Yet homophones can turn nasty, thanks to the two-step process needed to reach the solution. Unlike anagrams, where mixing letters will unveil your answer, the homophone variety expects you to find a synonym, utter that synonym, and that way hear your solution across

E X A M P L E S

Homophone

1. *Small area of land, I'll say* (4) [Henry Hook]
2. *Shopkeeper pronouncedly less refined* (6) [Rufus]
3. *Broadcast praises English cricket ground* (5) [DA]
4. *Extent of audible moans* (4) [Quantum]
5. *Just a pioneer aviator in the air?* (5) [DA]
6. *Wants to sound negligent* (5) [Rufus]
7. *Fabric noisily moved back and forth* (5) [Henry Hook]
8. *Fool appearing busier, we hear* (5) [Paul]

ANSWERS: 1. ISLE (sounds like I'll), **2.** GROCER (grosser), **3.** LORDS (lauds), **4.** SIZE (sighs), **5.** RIGHT (Wright), **6.** LACKS (lax), **7.** SUEDE (swayed), **8.** MORON (more on)

the airwaves. It is no surprise then, looking back at my tube-trial, my average success time when grappling with audio-clues was marginally slower than the mix-and-make variety of anagrams: most likely the difference between one step and two.

Cranking up the difficulty a few degrees, the two-step dance of homophone clues can also gain a tripping point, involving a second word to utter. To hear the twist for yourself, consider Mudd's booby trap below. Instead of one word to vocalise, this clue entails an acoustic version of charades, where the answer is the upshot of two audio-bits aligned in sequence:

Diatribe, outspoken Siamese attack? (6)

Outspoken is the signpost, a nudge towards the sonic realm. Sure enough, the moment you utter Thai (*Siamese*) and raid (*attack*), you'll hear the missing match for diatribe: TIRADE. 'Thyme' now for your own hearing check, with the final clue in the Homophone Examples box another double-bunger, much like Mudd's Thai-raid.

Containers

Otherwise known as sandwich clues, the container recipe is a popular device. To see how they operate, notice how OPERATE is ORATE around PE, just as JUST is S sandwiched by JUT. Did you see how I changed the emphasis in those examples? Simple as it sounds, you need to keep in mind that OPERATE can entail ORATE around PE—or can see PE occupy ORATE.

Seems a superficial difference, but the choice of description is critical when tackling containers. Solvers must BEWARE a BEE can fly around WAR, or WAR may interrupt BEE, with either scenario delivering BEWARE. Put another way, X can sit in Y, just as Y can hold X, leading to the same result. So long as you follow the clue's instructions—inserting or embracing—you'll arrive at a solution that resembles a nest of two words to make a new word.

Bearing these two modes in mind, the container clue recruits one of two signpost styles. If *containment* is the mode, then look for words suggesting holding or nursing. And if *insertion* is the game, then seize such signs as amid or among, breaking or filling. (The boxes on pages 117 and 118 list more.)

To give you a taste of both recipes, let's look at two clues. Here's the first sample, served up by Firefly, a setter with London's *Telegraph*:

Maiden's in stupor with punctuation mark (5)

Firefly employs the most popular signpost in the container racket—the all-time favourite of *in*. Remember, when you see *in*, suspect insertion.

To translate the clue into plain English, when you put *maiden* inside a word for *stupor*, you fashion a *punctuation mark*. (Keep in mind that back in the Charades segment women could be abbreviated into W, as per the powder-room door.) By the same token, cricket fans will tell you that a maiden—a bowler's over that produces no runs—is commonly reduced to M.

Yes, this shorthand language is a feature of cryptic puzzling, enabling a setter to say a lot with very few words. Soon, before the abbrevs run rampant here, I will be looking at the common candidates used to denote a single letter. (See the Deletions segment for more.) But let's get back to Firefly's stupefied maiden while the iron is hot.

In so many words, what punctuation mark—the likely definition on display—has five letters, including an M. Even handier, what four-letter word for stupor can M occupy to help spell that missing mark?

CO[M]MA, of course. The clue is a golden example of the insertion command, where X goes into YY to create Y[X]Y.

The equation is again reflected in a *Times* construction, puzzle 11,123:

Pick up article in valley = GLE[A]N

Yet gleaning this style of container clue is only half the story. We need to see the other equation at work, such as in this clue by Busman, another UK *Telegraph* compiler:

Mole embraced single early settler (7)

S I G N P O S T S

CONTAINER: HOLDING (a sampling)

about	embrace	over
absorbing	encompass	pen
accept	engulf	pinch
accommodate	entertain	pocket
admit	envelope	possessed
adopting	fencing	protect
around	flanks	restrict
assuming	frame	robe
astride	gathering	round
ate	getting around	sandwiches
bags	gobble	screen
bandage	grab	seal
blanket	grasp	securing
bottles	gripping	seize
bound	harbour	shackle
boxing	hedge	shelter
cake	hold	skirt
capture	host	snare
carry	house	stifle
circle	home to	stocking
clasp	hug	store
clothes	including	suck in
clutch	inspire	surround
collected	jacket	swallow
coming to grips with	keep	taking in
couch	make a case for	touring
cover	mask	trap
detain	netting	welcome
drink	outline	without
eat	outstanding	wrap

(Busman is an alias of Tom Johnson, whose love for Malta's esoteric bus-fleet provides his by-line. The same man is also Gozo—named for a Maltese town—in the *Financial Times* and Doc in *The Independent*, honouring a wordier namesake, the dictionary pioneer Samuel Johnson.) Sorry, let's refocus on his clue:

`S` `I` `G` `N` `P` `O` `S` `T` `S`

CONTAINER: BEING HELD (a sampling)

access	fit	opening
board	fit into	parks in
boards	get [stuck] into	parting
boring	impede	plug
boxing	in detention	resident in
breaks	introduced to	stuffing
come into	introducing	tuck into
cracking	invested	tunnels
don	laid into	visit
feeding	lines	visit/ing

CONTAINER EXTRA

Occasionally the container clue can play poetic, implying the act of cloaking (or being cloaked) by hijacking a common word or expression. For instance, any word or phrase starting with IN—such as INSTEAD, INDEED or IN CASE—could be enlisted for the task, though not always stated. As a foretaste:

Angry with me as a substitute? (7) = STEA[ME]D (me in-stead)

Wilier still, container clues could *imply* clothing or encasing, such as another homegrown clue:

Celebrate Oz dog, formally? (2,2,4) = GO[TOTO]WN (Toto in gown)

Rest assured, such constructions are rare. Nevertheless, it pays to put the more lyrical container clue on your watchlist.

Mole embraced single early settler (7)

To an experienced eye, the most telling word is *embraced*, that mainstay of container clues, where the ocean is engulfing the fish rather than the fish being in the ocean.

If that instinct is right, then a word for mole is embracing a word for single, the whole caboodle a synonym for an early settler.

See how I've sliced the clue for you? Tossing up between *single early* and *early settler*, the latter is more logical and the likelier definition, as long as *embraced* sits amid the wordplay's container instructions. The clue can be parsed this way:

Mole around single = early settler

Swap each of those three elements for synonyms, and you're moments from boarding Busman's chicanery. The answer, a synonym for early settler, in fact appeared a few paragraphs back, in reference to wordsmith Samuel Johnson.

Mole is neither a blemish, digger nor spy, but a structure extending into the water. Sure enough, build PIER around a word for *single*, and there you have it: PI[ONE]ER.

Now it's your turn to get stuck into the next eight samples, a medley that commands you to insert as well as enwrap.

E	X	A	M	P	L	E	S							

Container

1. *Empty container found outside prison* (6) [Quantum]
2. *Complimented Fred drinking milky coffee* (9) [DA]
3. *Catches held in actual practice* (9) [Columba]
4. *Damp fog conceals nothing* (5) [Henry Hook]
5. *Keen to have creative work around office* (6) [Mudd]
6. *Married nursing assistant had babies* (7) [Arachne]
7. *Fight is eclipsed by all others* (6) [Nutmeg]
8. *Intrudes in health resort, breaking locks* (10) [Gila]

ANSWERS: 1. VA[CAN]T, **2.** FLAT[TE]RED, **3.** RE[HEARS]AL, **4.** M[O]IST, **5.** AR[DEN]T, **6.** W[HELP]ED, **7.** RES[IS]T, **8.** TRE[SPA]SSES

Hiddens

You deserve a break, after breaking words down, uttering Indian cities, immersing maidens into comas. How's the pulse rate? That was a lot of mental gymnastics in a few short pages, especially if you're new to the sport. By way of relief—and reward—let's meet the simplest recipe in the book. I've saved this as a deliberate pick-me-up, to give you a second wind.

It's a bizarre story, but the so-called hidden formula delivers the answer intact, just as *bizarre story* hides ARREST and a LAD snoozes in *formula delivers*. The main challenge (which holds INCH) in solving a hidden clue is realising it's a hidden clue. The moment you do, the solution is there in plain sight.

Helping you to make that discovery will be a signpost implying contraband, a nod towards the secret length of language being smuggled within the clue. See the box for the common indicators, including the most common trio of some, part and partly—plus the fourth musketeer, of.

For example, a clue from the late Yorkshire poet, Harold Massingham, better known to solvers as Mass in *The Independent*:

A creature of malevolence (4)

WOLF, maybe. CROC or ORCA also spring to mind. Or possibly BEAR or YETI, if your brain is locked into the literal. Whereas a cryptic thinker will start digging, looking at the letters of *malevolence*, burrowing for the answer like a VOLE.

It's easy when you know how, which is why hiddens can torment. Of all the recipes, this black duck gives me the most grief, as I often overthink the ruse, looking for synonyms or anagrams when all the while the letters are on display, if I know where to look.

Like all other clue categories, the hidden mode does not squander a word. Every hidden clue entails three elements—definition, signpost and fodder (where the answer is covertly lying). Now and then the signpost and fodder can fuse, making this formula tougher to rumble,

| S | I | G | N | P | O | S | T | S | ■ | | | | | ■ | | | | ■ |

HIDDEN (a sampling)

a bit of	extract	part of
a little	feature	partial
a lot of	feeding	passage
array	fences	piece
assimilate	fragment	piece of
attributes	from	pocket/s
bottled by	gems	prisoners
bridge	harbour	resident
buried in	held by	sample
cake	held in	secretly
captive	hidden in	segment
central to	hostage	series
characters in	in	shackled by
components	in part	share
concealed by	join	show
constituents	letters from	shows
contained in	lodger	slice
content	nest	some
contributing to	not entirely	squirrels
elements of	not entirely visible	stuffing
encapsulating	of	train
essential to	owned	within
essentially	part	

yet the principles remain inviolate. To illustrate that last point, here's one of mine:

Bed inscribed (4)

How can two words carry three elements? Simple—two of those elements have united. Thus CRIB (your missing *bed*) is *in/scribed*. Watch out for such stratagems, and see how you cope with these eight examples.

E	X	A	M	P	L	E	S							

Hidden

1. *Type of pop provided by band is corny* (5) [Shed]
2. *Lunched daring, consuming cheese* (7) [*Times* 10,786]
3. *Musical creation of Sullivan, The Mikado* (6) [Paul]
4. *Scary figure in gym on steroids* (7) [Qaos]
5. *Building doomed if icebound* (7) [DA]
6. *Apply a bit of simple mentoring* (9) [Hectence]
7. *In winter a liaison, amongst other things* (5,4) [Falcon]
8. *A bunch of pseudos of the art editor kind* (4-7) [Arachne]

ANSWERS: 1. DISCO, **2.** CHEDDAR, **3.** ANTHEM, **4.** MONSTER, **5.** EDIFICE, **6.** IMPLEMENT, **7.** INTER ALIA, **8.** SOFT-HEARTED.

Reversals

Back in 1989, Cher longed to turn back time, if she could find a way. Thanks to this next cryptic recipe, the pop diva needs look no further. In the reversal formula, turning back is the key, a method that makes AVID out of *diva making a comeback*, or *turns back time* into EMIT.

Signposts for a reversal include words like reflect or reflection, or anything implying a switch in direction, such as the box on pages 123–4 reveals. This is the recipe that celebrates the fluke of turning *tops* into SPOT, or that LAPTOPS arises from a capsized *spot-pal*.

That last gimmick highlights an added extra trick of solving this formula, as sometimes the answer may involve multiple words to switch. PINE NUT, for one, may hail from *tune* and *nip* or PINE GAP from *page* plus *nip*.

The other skulduggery to note is the answer's location in the grid. For Across clues, the signpost will range among recalling, retiring, recoiling and so on—any verb to suggest letters ebbing from right to left, or heading in a westerly direction. Meantime Down clues will carry an indicator to signal climbing, rising, turning up, travelling

S I G N P O S T S

REVERSAL: UP AND BACK (a sampling)

about	drawn up	keep back
all round	elevated	knock back
arising	elevation	laid-back
around	erect	left
ascend	escalating	lift
ascendant	flip	lifted
ascending	flipped	lifts
back	flipping	looking back
back-to-front	from below	looking up
backfiring	from the bottom	make a comeback
backing	from Down Under	mounted
backslide	from the south	moved up
backtrack	go around	northbound
backward	go back	on the contrary
boomerangs	go round	over
bring back	go west	overthrow
bring up	going back	overturn
brought about	going north	overturned
brought up	going round	perversely
building	going up	picked up
capsized	head over heels	pivot
cast up	held up	promoted
clambered	hiking	put up
climbing	hoisted	raised
climbing up	hold up	raising
come about	in circulation	rear
come back	in lift	rebuffed
come up	in recession/	recall
comeuppance	retirement	recalled
coming back	in retrospect	recede
coming up	in return	recess
contrary	in turn	recoil
counter	inversion	recurrent
cutback	invert	reflect
cycle	keel over	reflection

regress	rose	turn back
reject	rotate	turn over
repulsed	round	turn up
retire	scaling	turned
retired	send up	turning
retiring	sent back	turnover
retreat	sent up	turns
retreating	serve up	twisted
retrograde	set back	up
retrospective	set up	up-and-coming
return	setback	upended
reversal	shoot up	uplift
reverse	shown up	uplifting
reversed	soars	uprising
reversing	spun	upset
reversion	stuck up	upside down
reverted	subversion	upstanding
review	suffer setback	upturn
revolution	switch	upward
revolutionary	take up	used up
rise	the wrong way	withdraw
rising	topsy-turvy	written up
rolling	turn	

north. Thus the signpost honours the motion within the diagram, whether the horizontal entry is moving back, or the vertical entry is travelling up.

Let's meet one of each type to grasp the reverse gear. Firstly, an Across answer from veteran ocean sailor and compiler Gaff (alias Peter Willmot) in the *Financial Times*:

> *Sign that clownfish is back* (4)

Finding the answer is a cinch if you consider *Finding Nemo*, the Pixar hit of 2003. But wait, is your answer NEMO, or the fish's backwards cousin OMEN? Look at Gaff's clue—the wording is telling you. The *clownfish is back* to create the *sign*—OMEN is your answer.

Turning our attention to a Down clue, you'll notice my signpost takes a turn upwards:

Explosive or metal upended? (5)

Question: what's the smallest metal name in the periodic table, even before considering symbols? It's TIN, while OR-TIN (*or metal*) when *upended* makes the *explosive* NITRO. Kaboom!

Thinking outside the square is tough enough without thinking backwards outside the square, right? Don't sweat. Reversal clues can be treacherous for a rookie to undo, but at least the formula's signposts are reasonably clear, whichever way they point. Get that far, and the letters in the grid will help you see the right direction. That way you'll discover an uprooted *yam* is MAY, while a *golf* setback is a FLOG. Time for your turn, with the last three clues entailing double-twists.

E	X	A	M	P	L	E	S								

Reversal

1. *Smack insect from behind* (4) [*Times* 10,833]
2. *Hamsters, perhaps, pace about* (4) [Arachne]
3. *Boat in waters going west* (5) [Henry Hook]
4. *Record reviewed for UK college* (4) [Tramp]
5. *Turn sack into puppet* (4) [Columba]
6. *Boy's limb in lift* (5) [DA]
7. *Talk softly, overturning odds?* (6) [Emily Cox & Henry Rathvon]
8. *Mining district turns back Bedouin on border* (7) [DA]

ANSWERS: 1. TANG<, 2. PETS<, 3. SLOOP<, 4. ETON<, 5. TOOL<, 6. NI+GEL<, 7. MUR+MUR<, 8. PIL<+BARA<

Deletions

When *Oliver* loses face he produces LIVER. And when he fails to finish, the boy transforms into OLIVE. Or, when a H-dropping Cockney utters *Harrow*, a posh part of London, you end up with ARROW.

So goes the deletion formula, the last of the eight principal recipes. The key is clipping off a letter or more to fashion the solution. Sometimes that paring can be up the front, so *learning* graduates into EARNING. Or sometimes the bottom is scratched, so to speak, and *Homer* turns into HOME.

Note, there's no mixing involved. It's all about cherry-picking one piece from the pie, or picking out *ce* from *piece* to make PIE. Even DELETION can be viewed as a depleted version of *depletion*, losing its *p*—since subtractions can occur within a word's midriff as often as either end. By the same measure, *delectation* or *delegation* can be reduced to DELETION when some central letters are removed.

Such an operation introduces a few new things to consider. The first is the probable array of deletion markers (see the signpost boxes on pages 127–8), while the second idea is called cryptic shorthand, the sort of sleight we've met before. Remember back in the Charades segment, when women led to W, as per the toilet symbol? Just as maiden was cryptic-code for M?

Deletion clues draw heavily on such ruses. To render ELATION from *relation* you need to remove its initial *r*. Often a setter will indicate this snip by saying things like topless or faceless, heading off or initially lost.

The other option is referring to that R in particular, calling on cryptic language to imply a single letter. R, in this case, can be denoted by river or Republican, right or resistance (as in physics), even rook and runs (from chess and cricket respectively). This may seem a bit of a stretch, but many of these codewords recur, giving you a chance to get fluent in the dialect. Check the abbreviations boxes on pages 129–31 and you'll soon get familiar with this secret cryptic alphabet.

S I G N P O S T S

DELETION: FIRST LETTER (a sampling)

after facelift	fail to start	needs no intro-
bar opening	first to go	duction
behead	guillotine	scratch head
blow top	headless	skimmed
bow out	initiated	topless
defaced	leaderless	topping
discovered	lead-free	tops
doff cap/hat	lost at The Front	veneer removed
dropping head	masking face	wipe brow

S I G N P O S T S

DELETION: LAST LETTER (a sampling)

abbreviated	docked	missing final
all but	dropping behind	mostly
almost	endless	nearly
back away from	*Footloose*	no closer to
backdrops	going short	no end of
baseless	inadequate	one shy
briefly	incomplete	scratching bottom
clipped	last to quit	shortly
contracted	lose footing	tip off
cropped	Manx (no tail)	virtually

S I G N P O S T S

DELETION: MIDDLE OR CONTENTS (a sampling)

after vacation	gutless	pitted
content to go	heartless	scratching belly
discontented	hollow	unfulfilled
disheartened	knocking stuffing out of	unpacked
empty	lose focus	vacant
evacuated	not content	vacuous

| S | I | G | N | P | O | S | T | S | ■ | | | | ■ | | | | ■ |

DELETION: SIDES (a sampling)

exposed	not taking sides	side-splitting
fleeced	off-limits	skinned
naked	peeled	unrestricted
no-frills	shelled	unwrapped

Of course, a setter can turn creative too, straying from the shorthand staples to signify any given letter. Keeping with R, here's a dozen other ways the letter might be singled out:

airbase (base of air)

computer terminal ('terminating' letter of computer)

Labor backing (the back of Labor)

lead to ruin

paperback

quarter-final (final letter of quarter)

rear end

restaurant starter

Romeo (from the phonetic alphabet used by radio operators)

rooftop

summer's close

tenderfoot

While this type of guile won't infest every puzzle, a rewired brain will be leery of such incognito indicators. *Pencil lead* may be graphite—or *p*. *Bigfoot* may mean sasquatch—or *g*.

Equipped as you'll ever be, let's see how you manage this deletion by *The Guardian*'s Arachne, alias Sarah Hayes, a former lecturer in Russian at Manchester University:

Gas in technical language, ignored at first (5)

Lecturers generally use technical language, the kind that bewilders the outsider. Can you name this particular lingo? And, going one step further, can you ignore that word's first letter to reveal a gas?

The gas is inert, unlike your neurons right now. If they fire well, you'll soon pounce on j/ARGON as your element.

This next example, from the late Albie Fiore (better known as Satori in the *Financial Times*), sticks with the periodic table but plays a different trick. Not only do you need to delete an end letter, but that same deletion accompanies an untouched word to make your second mystery element:

Deadly stuff when bum's not quite pleasant (7)

The phrase *not quite* suggests falling short. A common synonym for *pleasant* is nice, and *not quite* nice is NIC. So we know the *deadly stuff* ends in those three letters, and begins with a synonym of *bum*.

COMMON ABBREVIATIONS (a sampling)

A   ace, ampere, answer, area, blood group, key, note

B   bachelor, billion(s), black, blood group, book, born, boron, bowled, British, bye, key, note

C   captain, carbon, caught, century, chapter, Charlie, clubs, cold, hundred, key, note

D   daughter, Delta, Democrat, diamonds, died, duke, five hundred, Germany, key, note

E   bearing, drug, east/ern, echo, ecstasy, energy, English, key, note, point, quarter, Spain

F   false, female, fluorine, following, forte, foxtrot, France, frequency, key, note

G   gallons, Germany, golf, good, grand, key, note

H   hard, hearts, height, helicopter, Henry, heroin, horse, hospital, hot, hotel, hour, husband, hydrogen

I   ego, India, iodine, island, one, single

J   jack, judge, Juliet

K   grand, kilo, knight, potassium, thousand

L   fifty, lake, learner, left, length, Lima, line, litre, pound

M   maiden, male, mark, married, mass, men, metres, Mike, mile, million, minutes, motorway, thousand

N   bearing, knight, name, neutral, new, nitrogen, noon, north/ern, November, point, Pole, quarter

O   circle, duck, hug, love, nothing, old, Oscar, ring, sign of affection, zero, zip

P   page, Papa, park, pass, pawn, penny, piano, power, pressure, quiet/ly

Q   Quebec, queen, question

R   king, radical, Republican, resistance, reverse, right, river, Romeo, rook, runs

S   bearing, point, Pole, quarter, second, sierra, singular, son, south/ern, spades, succeeded, sulphur

T   bone, model, shirt, tango, temperature, tense, time, ton, true

U   horseshoe, posh, turn, uniform, united, university, upper-class, uranium

V   against, chevron, five, verb, versus, very, Victor, volume

W   bearing, point, quarter, tungsten, week, weight, west/ern, whisky, wicket, wide, with, women

X   by, kiss, ten, times, unknown, vote, wrong

Y   unknown, Yankee, yard, year, yen

Z   unknown, Zulu

CRYPTIC ABBREVIATIONS (a sampling)

A   airhead, arrowhead, *Braveheart*, catgut, first of all, inner peace, lead to arrest, malcontents, middle man, Obama's right

B   baseball cap, bathing cap, being upfront, bulkhead, burying head, led to believe, Lib backing, first blood

C   coalface, commanding lead, copperhead, cotton top, head-on collision, lead in comedy

D   back of beyond, dead-end, defendant fronting, Delta, desktop, dog's lead, dunce's cap, end-to-end, godsend, *Howards End*, lead in drama, red caboose, rushed behind, third base, touched base, turned stern

E athlete's foot, back of Bourke, back of envelope, barefoot, become stern, close finish, dovetail, elected leader, electric lead, ending in haste, *fin-de-siecle*, home base, movie trailer, rearrange

F defender, defending, Family First, figurehead, *Firestarter*, flathead, traffic hub

G bigfoot, coming closer, dropping back, girl's left, KGB hub, legend, pig's arse, tight belly, touching base, wagtail

H approach from behind, cap in hand, end of epoch, hatchback, head of hair, head on pillow, heading for home, hilltop, hit head, touch base

I big heart, semifinal

J first of June/July, hook, jump-start

K back of truck, back-to-back, backpack, cocktail, kilo, kneecap, rock bottom, sharkfin, trick ending, weekend

L back from jail, discarded lace, fall back, head of lettuce, laptop, Liberal backing, naval base, startling, swollen belly

M end of term, film trailer, madcap, masthead, motormouth

N cottontail, end of autumn, fanbase, narrow opening

O apologist, boundless joy, cipher, himbo's bottom, Maroon 5, photo finish, so pointless

P airport hub, apple core, base camp, empty on the inside, epicentre, lead in play, pencil lead, person's debut

Q equal second, Qantas pilot

R airbase, backpacker, computer terminal, Labor backing, lead to ruin, mezzo-soprano, paperback, quarter-final, rainbow, raises head, rear end, restaurant starter, rooftop, silverback, summer's close, tenderfoot

S back in business, back to basics, ending in tears, gets behind, head of steam, inglorious end, origin of species, salary cap, Scarface, speed dial, spinning top, steel cap, touches base, transport hub

T back on diet, back-to-front, first base, heading for trouble, hotfoot, opening in traffic, tabletop, thin on top, tight finish, toecap, treetop, wit's end

U fruit core, hubbub, inside-out, shelled out, up-front, you texted

V centre of gravity, every second, lavender, violin bow

W last to know, network hub, rear window, waterfront, woollen top

X crossed lines, oxtail

Y army base, back from holiday, ending in disarray, piggyback, pussy-foot, sandy bottom, and Spanish, spy base, sticky end, Yankee

Z calzone filling, showbiz finale

Congratulations, you have extracted the poison. Better than that, ARSENIC represents your first hybrid clue, where Satori has combined a charade formula with a deletion, the chemical equation reading like so:

ARSE + NIC/e = ARSENIC

The next chapter, 'Guru yoga', will contort your neurons in extreme ways, getting you to regularly splice two formulas in the one clue. But let's not get ahead of the game, not when we have a set of deletion delights to enjoy.

E	X	A	M	P	L	E	S								

Deletion examples

1. *Her pa heads off for a time* (3) [Arachne]
2. *Endlessly hopeful for painkiller* (7) [Logodaedalus]
3. *Monastery not on for expertise* (7) [DA]
4. *German poet leaves without finishing article* (6) [Aelred]
5. *Fur supplier has head shaved precisely* (2,1,1) [Enigmatist]
6. *Heartless gaoler gets the bird* (6) [Mass]
7. *Space traveller wasted from ride skipping outskirts* (8) [DA]
8. *Wife leaving, got bigger cut* (4) [Nutmeg]

ANSWERS: 1. ERA [h/ER+p/A], 2. ASPIRIN/g, 3. M/on/ASTERY, 4. GOE/s+THE, 5. s/TOAT, 6. TUR/n/KEY, 7. ASTEROID [w/ASTE/d+f/RO/m+r/ID/e], 8. w/AXED

Bending the brain a little further

Toss the treadmill. Ditch the dumbbells. The tyro tutorial is done and dusted. Now we move into an agility session for the more advanced solver.

Curlier propositions, trickier posers—these next pages will turn your lobes inside-out, helping your imagination bend to the task of cracking the more evasive puzzles.

'Neuro-cardio', our start-up chapter, was your chance to establish a firm toehold in the climbing wall. But if you've been around the cryptic block a few times, then you won't be daunted by a standard anagram or a plain reversal. This coming workout is your invitation to advance your agility, attempting a rundown of rarer clue types, as well as a few insider hints into cryptic arts.

To begin, let's meet a tongue-tied priest from Oxford and the spoonerism.

Spoonerisms

WAYNE BRAVE is not a real person. Rather, he's a spoonerism of BRAINWAVE. Just as CANE BRANDY is no genuine liquor, but a mangle of BRAIN CANDY, those tasty treats that clues can be.

Both makeovers fall into the spoonerism basket. Take a second look to see how they work, if you don't know the foolery already. Named after Oxford's don of ethics, Reverend William Spooner, the wordplay relies on the switching of initial consonant(s). The poor old prof, holding tenure from 1867 until 1924, burbled stuff like pear spew when he meant spare pew, or calling Our Loving Shepherd a shoving leopard.

To make jaw yob (sorry, your job) a little easier, every cryptic clue involving this trick will almost always name-check Spooner himself, meaning this formula bears the most obvious flag of them all. As soon as you see the name Spooner, you can identify which words need transforming, and claw year. (Damn—you're clear.)

The only hitch is that few clues will give you those 'fodder words' verbatim. Like the following clue:

Film Spooner's lee cargo (3,5)

Whether you've seen *Key Largo* from 1948, or you've been to Key Largo off Florida—that doesn't matter. The clue does most of the work for you, telling you which words to finagle. All you have to do is follow the instructions.

Where the recipe gets more testing is when a synonym step is added. Reusing *Key Largo* as our answer, the revised clue might read:

Film Spooner's sheltered freight (3,5)

Freltered Shate is not a film, if we were to spoonerise the words presented. Hence you need to summon the right synonyms to enact the spoonerism. Homophone clues demand the same middle step—giving you the synonym of the word you ultimately need to voice.

Before we tackle a few spoonerism examples, mayor in bind (you know what I mean) that sometimes a single word can be the spoonerism's source—or answer. *Dutch town* yields TOUCHDOWN, inviting my clue:

Land in Rotterdam, according to Spooner (5,4) = TOUCH DOWN (spoonerising Dutch town)

In a similar vein, a single-word solution may hold spoonerism potential, such as this original:

Track two sea creatures for Spooner? (7) = RAILWAY (spoonerising WHALE/RAY)

Spelling is the other quirk worth observing. In every sample so far, the answers have made slight adjustments to honour the spoonerism's sound. To be technical, *lee cargo* makes CEE LARGO, yet that spelling disregards the hard *C* from *cargo*—hence KEY LARGO is the sonic outcome. Likewise *Dutch town* mutates into TOUCHDOWN, not TUTCHDOWN, erring on the side of existing words.

Gear hose!

E	X	A	M	P	L	E	S								

Spoonerism

1. *Spooner to label giant mammal as dainty bird* (7) [DA]
2. *Tinned sort of offal Spooner delivers in barrow* (8) [Hoskins]
3. *Not enough tarts for Spooner? Don't you believe it!* (4,2,4) [Crux]
4. *Fat cat Spooner's copies of* Playboy? (9) [Arachne]

ANSWERS: 1. WAGTAIL (spoonerising tag whale), **2.** HANDCART (canned heart), **3.** PACK OF LIES (lack of pies), **4.** MONEYBAGS (bunny mags)

Manipulations

As we've seen, spoonerisms swap opening consonants, turning *better locks* into LETTERBOX. This next formula pulls a matching stunt: swapping letters around, or switching letters within a word.

One way to imagine the formula is to picture a street magician switching cups on a table. The cups are opaque and upside-down. One cup hides a pea—the other four are empty. Your job as observer is to follow the pea. Whereas a solver's job is to try to see which letters are being swapped, turning TIRE out of TIER (switching the sequence of letters)—or TIRING out of TIMING (replacing a letter).

If that sounds brain-bruising, it can be. Manipulations rate among the tougher clues to unravel, their rarity a consolation.

A further consolation is the helpful language, presuming you know how to decode the clue—the clue's wording will lead you through the operation. Either a letter (or letters) will move within a word—changing *rarest* into ARREST, say—or an imported letter will arrive as replacement, seeing *rarest* mutate into RAWEST. Let's check out two examples, one for each kind of procedure, better known as the Switch and the Swap.

First, let's meet a sample from the Switch camp:

Waterbirds run, top to bottom (5)

Where's the signpost? Always ask that question. What's the clue telling me to do?

Rattle through a checklist if it helps, dismissing the likelihood of anagram (no sign of mixing), homophone (no sign of hearing), container (no sign of inserting, or holding), and so on.

Step by step you'll scratch most candidates, leaving you with the likely command *top to bottom*—a favoured expression in manipulations for reasons of seeming seamless.

To obey the command *top to bottom*, you must move the word's first letter to the end, move the top to the bottom as it were. Yet which word?

Look at the answer's length. We're seeking a five-letter synonym of *run*, with too many suspects to list easily. But a good crossword sleuth will suspect the word begins with S. Can you see why?

It's common sense: your solution is likely to be a variety of water bird, and we know most plurals end in S. Hence our run synonym will probably begin with S, the top letter destined to be the bottom, after the manipulation. A theory like this is a leap of logic, not faith. The more puzzles you confront, the more your mind will tease out such ideas.

Asked another way—what's a four-letter name for a waterbird? Four letters, as its plural form will make five. While GEESE is singular and plural without an S-bottom, those birds are the exception. All the rest pass muster: DUCK, SWAN, TERN, TEAL.

Try each bird out, adding an S to its head, seeing whether the masquerade produces a word meaning run: SDUCK (nup), SSWAN (a pale ship?), STERN (the ship's bottom?), STEAL (aaah . . .).

Hang on—does steal mean run? Kinda, sorta, but not really. If you steal my wallet, you might run away, but that's imprecise, and illegal. Now give it back.

A baseballer may steal a base, running from first to second, but again that's a stretch, and far less satisfying than scoot—

SCOOT? Try it out. Manipulate the top to the bottom—COOTS—and your bird is in the hand. A lot of fuss and flying feathers on the way, perhaps, but manipulations become smoother with practice.

So much for the switch formula, essentially a subtler means of performing an anagram. But what does the Swap procedure look like, the second style of manipulation? Take a gander:

Lying airhead in clique falls for one (7)

Airhead could be A—the head of air. We learnt that cryptic code in the last section, as part of the deletion game. Meantime *one*, the final word, is often shorthand for I.

Here in this clue we have an A falling for an I, the first letter succumbing to the second. But in what? Read the clue—it tells you. To make the message clearer, I've translated the cryptic-speak to help you see the game at large:

Lying [A] in clique falls for [I] (7)

Know any words meaning *clique*? Your suspect has seven letters, including an A, just as the clue spells out. As a bonus hint, let's turn

---

E	X	A	M	P	L	E	S							

Manipulation

Two of these clues involve a switch, while two entail a swap, replacing one letter for an import. If you followed our FACTION of COOTS, you'll intuit which is which.

1. *Parasites cling, first to last* (5) [*Times* 10,875]
2. *What is replacing a card game?* (5) [DA]
3. *Prison caused change of heart—that's the aim* (4) [Neo]
4. *After sex change, cleavage becomes goal* (7) [Donk]

ANSWERS: 1. TICKS (switch first to last in STICK), 2. WHIST (swap IS for the A in WHAT), 3. GOAL (switch inner pair of GAOL), 4. MISSION (swap F of FISSION for M—female for male)

to the master of techno-thrillers, Tom Clancy, who said, 'The difference between fiction and reality? Fiction has to make sense.'

True. Fiction is a fancy word for 'not true', the stuff of imagination. In short, lying. And FICTION is also the result of FACTION's A falling for I.

There's no question—these are tough clues to read, ten times harder than a Clancy thriller, but the more you grapple with the swapping and switching, the quicker your eye will follow the moving P—so to speak—under the magician's cups.

Codes

Who needs John Le Carré when cryptic crosswords offer all the code-breaking fun you'll ever need? Codes are clues whose answers are laced in their own wording, requiring you to pluck out selected letters to create the solution. Such clues may read this way:

Starters in race are motivated about doing athletics naturally fast (7)

Ignore the runners implied in the story. By now you should be wise enough to see through the clue and examine the words. Rather than sprinters, *starters* are initial letters, the seven letters starting the words in the following: *race are motivated about doing athletics naturally.* Together, what do the letters spell? The final hint is the clue's finish: *fast.*

Again, it's nothing to do with track and field, as the story is trying to suggest, but fast of a different stripe. Usually across May and June a faithful Muslim will observe RAMADAN, a fast of thirty days or so.

Other signposts which imply initial letters include fronts, faces, openers—and initially. When it comes to recognising recipe markers, many of the signposts listed in the Deletions segment can apply here. The difference gets down to process. While code-solvers must handpick letters to spell the answer, the deletion challenge depends on leaving the right leftover, once those letters have been removed.

In the meantime, other signpost variations can point you to letters in different positions, like in this clue from Gila, a compiler for *The Independent*:

Too many gluttons ask for seconds (4)

So persuasive is the story, it's hard to isolate the junction between wordplay and definition, or in this case: definition/wordplay. Almost invisible, the answer's synonym is standing at the head of the line: *too*. (Never overlook any word in any clue—remember that.) Going with *too* as definition then, we can now break the clue this way:

Too / many gluttons ask for seconds (4)

Spot the signpost? Rather than starters this time, Gila is telling you to consider the second letters in *many gluttons ask for*.

Codes can ALSO focus on the tail-enders, the wooden spooners, the lucky lasts, such as in this clue:

The solemn creed we worshipped lasts through (5)

Just like *too* in the last sample, *through* is easy to disregard. But beware—inconspicuous words are given their low profile for a reason, all the better to mislead the rookie. A synonym of *through* is ENDED, the lasts of the first five words: *The solemn creed we worshipped*.

Firsts, seconds, lasts—you've seen the gamut of the code genre. Now run the gauntlet.

E	X	A	M	P	L	E	S							

Code
1. *Foremost in the arts, painter is never granting audition* (6) [DA]
2. *Diners out, usually booking table, first of all making reservation* (5) [Times 10,774]
3. *Truck found behind rental limo over major highway* (5) [DA]
4. *Bottom line that's reduced flight fares by thirds* (5) [DA]

ANSWERS: 1. TAPING, 2. DOUBT, 3. LORRY, 4. NADIR

Alternations

A code of sorts, the alternation formula selects every odd or even letter from a clue's wording. OWL, for example, is nesting in the odd letters of ORWELL, or the even letters of BOSWELL, another English author. That cute fluke helps a setter create a clue like the following.

Hundred Acre Wood character oddly created by Orwell (3)

Evenly and *oddly* are common signals of the game, though the beacon you'd be wise to remember is *regularly*—as in the regular pattern of alternate letters, whether they're the odd or even letters. In a similar vein, *regulars* is also a regular offender, the very culprit in this sample:

Diehard regulars no more (4)

Bizarre, right? The regular letters of *Diehard*, the odds in this case, spell DEAD. That irony is right up there with *barbarian* oddly declaring BRAIN, or *blackberry*—the produce sold by greengrocers—rendering BAKER.

If not appearing as a whole recipe, the alternation trick can frequently appear to provide a letter-string that forms part of the solution. A case in point:

Polo regulars nibbled meal = PLATE

Or this one from Puck in *The Guardian*:

Language coming from Jack and Vera, regularly (4)

The mystery language here is also an island that doesn't speak this language. If that sounds like nonsense, then let's unpeel the cryptic language. *Jack* is J, as any cardsharp knows. Next are the words *and Vera*. (Newcomers would be forgiven for overlooking *and*, the conjunction next to invisible in common prose.) Select the regular letters of ANDVERA and you make AVA, which, when escorted by J, becomes the computer *language* JAVA, your solution.

Beyond the regular use of *regularly*, be cautious of any adverb suggesting now and then, such as *sporadically* or *intermittently*. More signpost suspects appear in the box below, as well as these examples here. See how many you can get right.

E X A M P L E S

Alternation

1. *Unique all-rounder regularly missed* (5) [Vlad]
2. *Message in bottle oddly missing* (4) [*Times* 10,816]
3. *Woman using handbag every so often* (3) [*Times* 10,860]
4. *Be married, failing intermittently* (3) [DA]
5. *Pocket needs repairing regularly* (4) [*Times* 10,050]

ANSWERS: 1. ALONE, 2. NOTE, 3. ADA, 4. ARE, 5. EARN

S I G N P O S T S

ALTERNATION (a sampling)

at intervals	not even	off and on
at odds with	now and then	periodical
evens out	occasionally	regularly
here and there	oddly	sporadic
intermittent(ly)	oddly deficient	

Puns

Become a crossword solver—it's a rewording career!
Zorro was a regular letter-writer.
Stiletto heels are archenemies.
Audiobooks are speaking volumes.

However cornball or twisted, all the samples above might be adopted by a playful setter. (And I don't mean a frisky puppy.) The first example deliberately tweaks a word into a pun—turning rewarding into rewording—while the others are capricious ways of defining the key word or phrase.

In American-style puzzles, which are separate from the cryptic genre, offering a range of quick and trivia clues, the occasional pun clue is called a daffy definition. My opening wisecracks are in that style, where wordplay acts as a comical description. (And if you recall, we tackled Joon Pahk's daffy clue back in Part One, where CAROL was *Number of holidays*.) Check out this trio, drawn from a single *New York Times* puzzle by veteran stylist Patrick Berry:

It's played close to the chest = UKULELE
People get off on them = EXIT RAMPS
Chain attached to buckets = KFC

All these clues belong under the same punbrella. Apologies in advance—this section is scattered with a father lode of Dad jokes, from COLDPLAY (*the Winter Olympics*) to ATHEISTS (*non-parishables*). Pun clues skew the language to smoke-screen the solution, although they promise a smile once the smoke clears. Indeed, in some British circles, the pun clue is dubbed an oblique or cryptic definition, making your role as solver a matter of realigning the language to match with dictionary-speak. to convert *Raspberry producer?* (say) into 'an organ that produces a raspberry effect', namely TONGUE.

Among cryptic clues, puns are often flagged by a question mark, your signal to uncover the potential mischief of the clue's wording. *Present day?* is a fresh way to see CHRISTMAS. Just as TOILET might be the *Place to go?* Or, *Sitting room?*

The other pun signpost can be brevity. This stands to reason, since wordplay and definition may be rolled into one. *Love handles* (the clue) could be fleshed into TERMS OF ENDEARMENT, the answer as payoff, lending sense to the pun. See how you go with this gem from the *Sunday Times*:

One shy of seven? (7)

Logic dictates the answer is SIX, but the answer's number of letters doesn't allow it. And besides, logic needs to step aside when a question mark comes along. Ration the rational—this clue needs more playful brainwork.

If I told you the answer starts with B and ends on L, does that help? Pun clues may rely on a few cross-letters in the grid to steer your thinking. Can you nominate a seven-letter word starting with B that means *shy*?

Please, don't be bashful. In fact, get happy with these four 'daffy definitions' to prove you're not sleepy. I've even supplied the first and last letters of each answer, rather than the solution's length, just to stop you getting grumpy.

E	X	A	M	P	L	E	S								

Pun

1. *One who's been given a court order?* (S-D) [Notabilis]
2. *Big Brother of Marxism?* (G-O) [Araucaria]
3. *Leaves home?* (T-G) [DA]
4. *Happy he wasn't, but much blessed?* (S-Y) [*Times* 10,029]

ANSWERS: 1. SEED, 2. GROUCHO, 3. TEA BAG, 4. SNEEZY

P	U	N		B	O	X									

WHAT IDIOT?

What idiot called them voodoo dolls instead of idol threats?
What idiot called it a second marriage instead of a repair job?
What idiot called them cogs instead of ferrous wheels?
What idiot called it a fold-away tray instead of a periodic table?
What idiot called it a vet instead of a dogtor?
What idiot called it Qatar Airways instead of Air Qatar?
What idiot called it quoits and not game of throwns?
What idiot called them jet-skis versus boatercycles?
What idiot called him a stepdad instead of a faux pa?
What idiot called it a mugshot instead of a cellfie?

Rebuses

Stone motherless—slang for sloshed, or an emphatic way of saying you're last in a race—might also be depicted this way:

__ __ R B L E

See the reasoning? While WARBLE and BURBLE fit the pattern, so does MARBLE. Or here that's MARBLE without its MA, a fanciful way of suggesting *stone motherless*. If you're still confused, let me translate the GARBLE.

'*Rebus*' is Latin for 'by means of objects', as that is how this clue recipe works. Akin to a visual code, the rebus delivers the solution as hieroglyph, a set of symbols you need to decipher. Notably, most rebus clues, such as our opener, don't accompany a definition, the answer instead being outlined 'by means of objects'.

Perhaps the most clichéd example of a cryptic rebus is GSGE, or *scrambled eggs*, a few steps ahead of the other clue people like to cite as cryptic thinking:

H I J K L M N O (5)

I'm presuming you know the gag already. This rebus is older than Pliny the Elder, producing WATER, or H to O.

Strictly speaking, however, clues like these last two are unlikely to appear in mainstream crosswords, as the rebus recipe is deemed a little *too* playful for most mastheads. Chances are, if a rebus does bob up, the symbol play will adjoin the answer's definition as well, such as this innovative gem from *The Times*:

Aim cryptically for something quite special = ONE IN A MILLION

Even with the solution, can you unlock the clue's deception? What if I rejigged the example to isolate the trick?

AIM, expressed cryptically, means something quite special

Million, the word, is usually abbreviated to M in newspaper headlines and articles. Therefore *aim* is one in a million, if you view the word through a cryptic lens.

A pure rebus might only offer *aim* as the clue—and nothing else. Or sometimes capital letters are used to bring the encoded word or cluster into sharper focus. This same play can go towards compensating for the definition's absence, as can occur in the rebus mode, although that scorns the rulebook in the eyes of most editors.

Nonetheless, a good rebus will oblige your brain to think outside the box. That last phrase in fact—THINK OUTSIDE THE BOX—was the solution for Tramp's ingenious rebus from a *Guardian* puzzle in 2011:

MUST'VE (5,7,3,3)

Get the cunning? It's hard to dismantle, but once you spot TV—or, the box—lodged inside MUSE, another word for think, the brilliance strikes you.

More typically, the rebus escorts a definition, unless the trick can extract both rabbits, such as this oldie from my own drawing board:

HERO? (4,4)

Yes, that darker font is deliberate. Why? Because BOLD TYPE, your answer, describes the typography as much as the personality of the fearless protagonist.

If the recipe feels a little flaky, then rest assured it's rare. Indeed, you're more likely to encounter the ruse in a cryptic answer, as seen here:

Haters the result of such sad cases? = BROKEN HEARTS

Follow the logic this time? The wording implies the rebus-logic of *haters* deriving from HEARTS when broken. It's a basic anagram when all is said and done, but a lot more evasive when your brain needs to infer the missing step. Keeping things on a cardiac theme, here's another rebus-flavoured clue:

Lover suggesting wee? (10)

So babe, know another word for lover? Or darling, what term of endearment could double as a cryptic indicator for WEE?

SWEETHEART is the missing label, hotcakes. Watch out for this inverted brand of rebus, which often uses words like *suggest* or *result*, and almost always carries a question mark. Like this one, from *Times* puzzle 11,123:

Al suggesting this department for customer service? (4,6)

If the crossword was quick, you'd be searching for a customer-service department. But since it's cryptic, you also can deduce that AL is the lateral outcome of the missing phrase, the middle of the four-letter word in fact. Indeed, AL is the centre of CALL, which is to say CALL CENTRE, a place for customer service: your answer.

Without resorting to customer service, or the help desk, see how you fare with these rebus samples. Before you begin, notice how no clue carries any upper-case words or clusters, a quirk more common to the solo rebus, with no accompanying definition. (This also suggests, as tough as these four samples are, that there is a definition escorting each rebus ruse.) Did I say tough? I'd rate the last two as difficult, extremely difficult when you have no cross-letters to assist.

E	X	A	M	P	L	E	S									

Rebus

1. *As cryptically suggested by this conflicted region* (6,4) [*Times* 10,853]
2. *Hear Ted is distraught?* (6-7) [*Sunday Times* 1004]
3. *Take in?* (4-4) [*Times* 10,638]
4. *How eagle's made descent* (7) [Donk]

ANSWERS: 1. MIDDLE EAST, **2.** BROKEN-HEARTED (and I even warned you about this), **3.** HALF-INCH, **4.** L/IN/EAGE

Punctuation

Now's the time to shelve the recipe book to issue a general warning. To paraphrase *Star Trek*, the cryptic crossword uses punctuation, but not as we know it. Be alert when it comes to hyphens, dots and squiggles on the puzzle page. Just as no word is wasted, no punctuation is either.

But rather than scare you with random caveats, let's take a peek at the various roles of punctuation in a cryptic habitat, just to see what you need to anticipate.

Telling the story

The surface sense is how smoothly a clue reads. The best clues tell their lie well, sucking you into the story while concealing the deeper truth.

Notice the comma in that last sentence? That's there because I extended my remark with an additional clause, enlisting a comma to annex the principal remark. It's simple enough, since that's how punctuation works in the real world. Compare that to Hazard's clue from *The Guardian*:

New woman, right? No way! (5)

There are three punctuation marks in one small bundle: comma, question mark, exclamation mark. Together the devices capture the clue's cadence, as if a flabbergasted speaker is responsible for the words, not a compiler. Say the clue aloud and you can almost imagine a person denying rumours of a new girlfriend in his life. Hazard is wanting you to think that way—to fall for the fiction—when really you can ignore the three bits of punctuation and read it as:

New woman right no way

To decrypt the clue, and get to the charade, you might even swap those marks you've dumped for symbols of a different kind:

New + woman + right = no way

New as in New Testament, or New South Wales, is often reduced to N, the letter. As for *woman*, who's the first female to spring to mind? There must be scores of girls' names of adequate length for this clue, yet the original suspect deserves to be EVE.

You know what comes next, right?

Wait, let's alter that punctuation to better reflect my meaning.

You know what comes next: right.

That's right, as in N+EVE+R = *no way*. Hazard's hazards are easier to surmount once you fleece the clue of its punctuation, converting the story into a cold equation.

When solving crosswords, you have to un-rut your brain that way, looking beyond your typical reading behaviour to expose the logic underneath. You may recall the words of linguist Debra Aarons, the academic we met in the chapter 'Dis/Connect': 'Once we view language, especially written language, as a string of elements, the play and puzzle possibilities are endless.'

To solve a cryptic puzzle, warn your neurons in advance. Instead of rational sentences, the stuff of essays and rental agreements, your grey matter will be dealing with deceptions, the sort that often rely on punctuation as their camouflage.

Symbol-minded

Then again, never ignore punctuation marks either. While trimming a clue to its bare bones may be useful, you're equally wise to question how each squiggle may contribute to the solution. Here's a clue I made a few years back:

Resembling: nudist camp? (6)

The question mark makes sense, lending an inquisitive lilt to the clue's story, but what is that colon doing?

If nothing is wasted, including punctuation, then what function does the colon fulfil? That question is pivotal.

Put it this way: if something resembling mist is misty, and something resembling fog is foggy, what word describes something colon-like? Ask Adam or Eve in their nudist COLONY.

Not only is the colon central to the clue, but the question mark is also meaningful, suggesting the wordplay has a playful result, combining the double-meaning formula with something of a pun.

And should nudity offend, here's one of Paul's clues from *The Guardian* that relies on clothing, and a vital piece of punctuation:

Style in T-shirt and Y-fronts, perhaps? (4)

Again, treat that question mark as a whimsy-warning. Pry deep into Paul's wardrobe for the joke to work. Here the recipe is the double definition, where a word for style is stitched within both garments.

What else do *T-shirts* and *Y-fronts* have in common? To the same list you can add a G-suit, a two-piece, a muu-muu and a ten-gallon hat. Spot the shenanigans now?

The answer is DASH, a synonym of style, as well as the punctuation mark. And should you quibble that the apparel names use a hyphen rather than a dash, keep in mind the question mark warns you of a looser interpretation.

Inner space

Part of the punctuation racket is the art of managing a clue's spacing. You can see that principle in action here:

'Partied awfully close,' I said (10)

Awfully is a common anagrind, or anagram indicator. Scramble those adjoining ten letters—CLOSEISAID—and you'll make a match for partied.

In this instance you should overlook the punctuation marks, as their main mission is camouflage—a bid to disguise the anagram fodder (*closeisaid*) by marking out space with the literary custom of quotation marks and the necessary comma. Strip it down, and *closeisaid*, when awfully handled, turns into SOCIALISED, or *partied*.

In this next example, you'll see how punctuation can arrange space in a different way. This gem is a dastardly construction from Philistine, another *Guardian* regular:

Booklet: What to do next (7)

Which path do you take here? Do you factor in the colon or give it the flick? If that dilemma was already dancing in your brain, then congratulations: you are one step closer to the inner cryptic circle.

Philistine's stealth lies in his use of compression, taking two words—*book* and *let*—and fusing them into a single entity. Of course you'd read *booklet* as booklet, rather than *book* (the definition) and *let* (the wordplay's first word). Why wouldn't you? That's what your brain is trained to do.

Yet cryptic language is a different beast, more novel than any novel. After years of hoovering up traditional prose, your frontal lobe needs to readjust, the better to prepare for this sort of trap, where setters can skip spacing or misleadingly add punctuation or chunk two elements into one misleading compound.

The answer to the clue is RESERVE. Can you see why? What if I added a bonus piece of punctuation to help out: RE-SERVE.

Tennis players will know the rigmarole of serving a let. That's where your service brushes the net-cord and drops to the other side. Presuming your ball lands in the service court, you get to serve again, or re-serve. Get it? *Booklet* is not booklet, but *book* (a verb meaning to reserve), and *let*, an invitation to serve twice.

To prove that kind of fusion can be a repeat offence, are you awake to Paul's chicanery from 2012?

Stimulating postcard? (8)

The obvious merger is postcard. So split the compound and reread the clue:

Stimulating post card? (8)

Note how that surface detracts from the original's fluency? This should help you see how a good compiler will exploit space—selecting or rejecting punctuation to make their trapdoor harder to detect.

Post has several meanings, from mail to job to mast. Another post found aboard a ship is the sail's strut, or spar. As for *card*, pick one from the deck. By this stage I'm hoping the answer is SPARKING your hippo campus. Sorry, hippocampus. This fusion fashion is all the rage.

Upcasing

Polish the European language is not to be confused with polish the shoe gunk. Well, it will be confused if the gunk—that is, the polish—starts a sentence and so appears as Polish. Crossword makers cherish that confusion. Pole the post and Pole the resident of Krakow are identical on the page if they're the first word of the clue.

The fancy tag for such words are capitonyms, an august band of rebels that includes turkey and August, tangier and May. Jack could be a candlestick-jumper, or a card, or a tyre-changing tool, just as a tyre could support a Ford, which happens to be a river-crossing when down-cased, while Tyre with a big T is an ancient port in Lebanon. You get the gist . . .

This next clue, courtesy of *The Guardian*'s Vlad, will test whether you have:

> *Robin and Batman initially arrested—crazy!* (9)

The exclamation mark is trying to sell the scandal of the clue's surface. Ignore it. Hoick the dash too—that's just more headline hype. Distil the clue to its essence, and look twice at *Robin*. Because it's coupled with *Batman*, you think superhero, right? An obvious conclusion, but remember that the laws of Cryptopia don't always mimic the real world's regulations. Pairing Robin with Batman is just your brain making a lazy union, leading your thoughts down the wrong pathway. Rather than the name, think the word. Think a bird, in fact.

Batman initially is B. The next word—*arrested*—has eight letters.

Make that nine when B joins the party. Now get crazy with that fodder, as the clue is urging, and see who or what flies out.

REDBREAST is the solution, beautifully disguised in the clue's syntax, promoting *robin* to the opening to make a crime-fighter out of the creature. Vlad's tweak could also act as a warning bell—usually it's Batman and Robin, but in this clue they're switched in order to upcase, ensuring the bird (*robin*) appeared as the caped crusader with his capital-R.

Not that syntax is the only means of introducing capitals. Sometimes a setter will 'upcase' a word within a clue just in the name of subterfuge. Take this example from *Times* puzzle 10,776:

The spirit of March and November (5)

Radio operators rely on the phonetic alphabet, where cops might read a partial numberplate SPF as Sierra Papa Foxtrot and Romeo and Juliet are often cryptic dialect for R and J.

Back to the *Times* clue, *November* is radio-speak for N, your answer's final letter, as that's the last detail supplied. So where can we find those other four letters to spell a spirit? Focus on *March*, but don't think the calendar. Downcase the M to make a parade of those 31 days, and the spirit may surface.

The *march* in question is a DEMO, which mutates into the *spirit* DEMON with *November* at its tail: a diabolical example of arbitrary upcasing.

Setters are shameless on this front. The classical setter Ximenes, deemed by many to have written the cryptic rulebook, addressed this in his 1966 bible, *Ximenes on the Art of the Crossword*: 'May one use a capital, where it isn't necessary, in order to deceive? May one abolish one, where it is, strictly speaking, needed, in order to deceive?'

What can I say? The man loved commas as much as rhetorical questions. But he did get around to answering his own moral dilemmas, his resolution no less punctuation-heavy:

'My answer to the first question is: Yes, at a pinch; but try, if you can, to put the word first in the clue or after a full stop in the course of it. My answer to the second question is: No! If you do abolish it, you aren't saying what you mean.'

Downcasing is therefore not a thing, not really. Don't expect to meet Hanks (the actor) appearing as hanks (the wool) within a clue. But the opposite is likely, where the balls of yarn are disguised as the *Forrest Gump* star, whether that word is opening the clue or not.

These are grounds, I hope, to be cautious of any clue's punctuation. Either you need to dismiss it entirely, or study it carefully, which sounds like Mad Hatter advice. Said another way: to crack the case, you need to look twice at letter-case, as well as dashes, brackets, colons and every other squiggle on the page, including . . .

Dot, dot, dot . . .

Beginners often pale at the sight of an open-ended clue, where a cluster of three dots seems to leave a clue in limbo. Like so:

A key part of cathedral . . . (5)

What's going on? What's the point behind the ellipsis, as those three dots are called? Ellipsis, in fact, stems from Greek, where '*elleipsis*' translates as 'omission'. Which invites the question: what has been omitted from the clue above?

In this case, nothing, because the clue is supposed to be viewed in tandem with its immediate successor, the next Across clue that reads like so:

. . . *partly collapsed* (4)

Huh? How can an ellipsis open a clue? The whole thing seems cruel and unusual. The quirk often serves to terrify rookies, but I need everyone to breathe easy. On the puzzle page the ellipsis has one of four functions, five if we count the standard literary function of ending a sentence in breathless suspense.

In cryptic clues, the first function of the ellipsis is to join two adjacent clues, like the examples above, which is a mode otherwise called a . . .

Shared definition

Compilers can be sneaky ratbags—and frugal too. Why waste ink giving the same definition twice when you can fuse two clues? That way the definition can be passed from one to the other like a relay baton. Let's browse those earlier examples again, this time reading them as a single unit:

A key part of cathedral . . . (5)

. . . *partly collapsed* (4)

Part of cathedral is the mutual definition, the so-called straight clue that satisfies either answer. That's why the phrase occupies the end of the first clue, the baton ready for the next clue to carry. Both your answers then will reveal two cathedral segments, but which ones?

The second clue is easier, thanks to the hidden signpost *partly*: tucked away in *collapsed* is APSE, a cathedral's recess.

So what about the first clue? Which piece of St Peters is implicated there? This time, instead of a hidden, the formula is a charade. *Key* is your key, a word that means many things, though here it is the geographical sense that comes to the rescue. Florida Keys, for one, is an archipelago of small islands, or isles, including Key Largo. Heeding the charade, A + ISLE = AISLE, another cathedral zone.

So there was nothing too hard about either clue, was there? The only thing to spook the rookie were those nasty dots. Unstitched, the two clues can be viewed like so:

A key part of cathedral (5)

Part of cathedral partly collapsed (4)

It's a piece of cake when you know how to interpret the ellipses. Here the overlap was a mutual definition, dovetailing two clues by virtue of their semantic coincidence. Which leads us to meet the punctuation's second function, where ellipses ask the solver to recycle an element of wordplay.

Shared wordplay

When a definition is mutual, the two paired clues will deliver related answers—the AISLE and APSE sort of duo. But when two clues share their wordplay element, the answers may be poles apart. Rather than shared semantics, the overlap may highlight a parallel piece of wordplay, a formula fluke that's signalled by the ellipses. Check out this pair:

Drop wrench . . . (4)
. . . and shout a great deal? (8)

The first clue calls on a double meaning, as two-word clues often will. Though of course, when the dots arrive, a solver can't be sure of either clue's precise length until both clues are parsed, and the overlap's been delineated. But by way of relief, here those two words—*drop wrench*—are the only words you need to pinpoint the answer.

Do you know a word that means both *drop* and *wrench*? As a friendly nudge, consider melancholia and agony: just your typical response to a crossword.

Saddened, your *drop* is prone to be a tear. Pronounced another way, a tear can also mean a painful sprain or *wrench*, making TEAR the first clue's answer.

But, just because the first clue enlists a double definition, doesn't mean its sibling will match that formula. Instead the second clue picks up *wrench* like a relay baton and uses the word as a signpost. Can you see how? *Wrench*, as you may already suspect, is a ready-made anagram pointer.

If that's the case, what needs wrenching? Your instincts should direct your gaze to the adjoining bunch of letters—eight in total, agreeing with the answer's length. Wrench ANDSHOUT, and you make a great deal.

The question mark warns you to take care—that maybe the definition is a little loose, a bit playful. And indeed a THOUSAND may amount to a great deal for some, but will be modest in other settings. Nonetheless, you've just met two clues that have shared a word (*wrench*), without sharing any parallels in their definition.

But just because they overlap in wordplay doesn't mean the clues own matching recipes. That's crucial to remember: when it comes to this style of splicing, the two clues can either belong to the same wordplay category or use a shared word—or words—in a different wordplay mode.

Did I mention the ellipsis can flag one of four cryptic modes? So far we've considered two, both of which mingle to make a third variety . . .

Alloy ellipsis

The name alone sounds alien, not a phrase you meet every day, nor will you meet too many alloy ellipses in your solving life either. As rare as nisil (an alloy of nickel and silver apparently), these clues fuse a wordplay element in one clue, with a definition element in the next—or vice versa.

So rare, we hardly need to spend a page on the oddity. But on the off-chance you bump into such an amalgam, and feel cheated that I never warned you, here we go:

Trusted new alloy . . . (5)
. . . *to nick, we hear* (5)

Alloy is the linchpin, the shared component fastening the clues together. In the first case, the word acts as anagram fodder. Treat those five letters anew and LOYAL arises, a synonym of *trusted*.

Moving on to clue 2, *alloy* deputises as the definition, ensuring this second clue is all wordplay. Here the formula is homophone, asking you to vocalise a word meaning *nick*. Pick the right synonym and you'll forge an alloy. Are you there yet? Or do you need a coffee to steel the nerves?

As I say, the combo is uncommon, but worth recording. An alloy ellipsis will operate like the last pairing, seeing a wordplay piece transpose into definition, or the opposite role-switching will occur, where one clue's definition mutates into an adjacent clue's mischief.

Three ellipses down—one to go. You'll be relieved to learn the last variety is more in keeping with language as you know it . . .

Grammatical grounds

DISCOVERY can be split into DISCO VERY, inviting a charade clue that may read this way:

Finding nightclub quite (9)

See the snag? As a clue that works, but as a story it sucks. Worse, the sentence is incomplete. 'Quite *what* . . . ?' you may well ask. The narrative is truncated.

Either a setter needs to recast her clue to fashion a smoother surface, or she can deploy the dots to spill her partial sentence into a rounder grammatical whole by linking it with the succeeding clue.

To illustrate this example, let's imagine the next clue's answer is EXAMPLE. Again the charade formula beckons, as EX-AMPLE offers neat possibilities. With a flick of the wrist, and a sprinkling of dots, one deficient clue can meld with another to read completely and coherently:

Finding nightclub quite . . . (9)
. . . old and spacious in illustration (7)

EX (*old*) and AMPLE (*spacious*) combine to make a word for illustration, bearing no relation to nightclubs except by virtue of sharing an ellipsis with its immediate neighbour, the two clues merging to build a stronger deception.

So the next time you encounter dots on the page, don't implode. The tool is a means of joining adjacent clues, depending on (a) their shared definition, (b) their shared wordplay element, or (c) the need to conjure a sleeker story. And that's that, unless . . .

&lits

I can't blame you for thinking the term &lit is some kind of rebus. What word opens with an ampersand anyway? If GRANDSTAND can be 'rebussed' into GR&ST&, then what might &lit represent?

The answer is the best clue possible. The duck's nuts. The cat's meow. The anchovy's elbows. Can you tell I'm excited? I love these clues. The term is short for 'and literally', and the &lit clue offers wordplay that *defines the answer as well*.

It seems a tall order, to combine both parts into one tidy clue, but that makes the joy all the more joyous whenever you can make the alchemy happen. Believe me, whenever I manage to pull off an &lit, I go do H&ST&& in the B&ST&.

Engineered just right, &lit clues can exploit any recipe we've met so far: charades, deletions, you name it. Anagrams are often implicated, such as this beauty:

Process promises a moth! (13)

The answer is a processed version of *promises a moth*. Rearrange those thirteen letters and you get METAMORPHOSIS—not just the upshot of the wordplay, but a concept the wordplay literally defines.

Keeping in that anagram groove, a compiler like Anax (alias Dean Mayer) devised this nifty &lit:

As ringtone that's swirling around?! (10)

You already know the formula involved. But which letters need mixing, and what will your answer mean? Being &lit, the clue is painting a complete picture, repurposing the wordplay to outline the solution.

Note the punctuation too—that comic-book coupling of ?!—with which &lit clues often end. Our first specimen didn't, of course, but most &lit clues do. A godsend in many ways, since this clue style can catch you off-guard, stirring two ingredients into one concoction.

As for the Anax clue, swirl around those ten opening letters—*as ringtone*—and you'll arrive at a word the entirety describes. I'd suggest you isolate the –ING suffix, keeping in line with the &lit's own case: *swirling around*.

We all know the scenario: stuck in a bus or trying to read in the library, general peace prevails until some bugger's mobile starts RESONATING throughout the space, as ringtones are wont to do.

The pure &lit avoids excess baggage, as seen in our initial samples. Every word has a role in both capacities, serving the definition as faithfully as the wordplay. However, there is a less pristine version, a modified &lit that may own a few excess frills for reasons of grammar or clarity. Elgar for *The Telegraph* composed one such clue:

Who has real relish in chaos? (4-6)

There's no exclamation mark this time, but you still need to bring your anagram A-game. The challenge here is to throw *real relish* into *chaos* to unmask someone who revels in bedlam. To soothe your brow I can tell you that's a HELL-RAISER.

Elgar's clue is elegant, though purists will argue it falls short of perfection since the wordplay (*real relish in chaos*) is accompanied by surplus words to mould the &lit trick into a question. Still lovely, but not as sumptuous as Paul's &lit, again banking on an anagram:

Order magnified with carbs?! (3,3,3,5)

Order is the ideal signpost, implying both a diner's request, as well as an edict to rearrange, so the wordplay is also the definition. Ordering *magnified carbs* will spell BIG MAC AND FRIES—no letter frittered!

Leaving anagrams alone, the &lit can resort to any recipe on the shelf, so long as the wordplay and definition are one and the same, the two elements bundled into one inseparable whole. Here's a glimpse of three charade formulas that reach &lit heights:

Wait, rear on jet, here? [*Times* 10,032] = BIDE+T
A choice of extremes in perversion?! [Paul] = P+OR+N
Oblivious to four notes? [*Times* 9793] = D+E+A+F

Even hiddens can join the party. This treat comes from Gaff in the *Financial Times*:

Sad is malcontent (6)

It's strange that a clue for DISMAL can be so delightful, noting how *content* can be both the emotion, and the cargo (so denoting the hidden formula). That's the rare bliss of &lit clues, where fate and finesse combine to forge one versatile unit: a piece of language that both defines and defiles its solution.

Knowing that any formula might lie under the &lit umbrella, see how many of these beautiful creatures you can decipher below.

E	X	A	M	P	L	E	S							

&lit

1. *Inclusion in 'Librettos' catalogue!* (5) [Henry Hook]
2. *Spot on head of India?* (5) [*Times* 10,876]
3. *A person gone idle? Nonsense!* (3-3,9) [DA]
4. *Outer part of some bud?* (5) [*Times* 10,929]
5. *Do this at risk of injury?!* (3,3,2) [DA]
6. *Who'd have role in alternative energy* (5,5) [Nestor]

ANSWERS: 1. TOSCA, 2. BIND+I, 3. OLDAGEPENSIONER*, 4. SE+PAL, 5. ASKFORIT*, 6. GREEN PARTY

[As you may recall, the asterisk marks the anagram mode.]

Hybrids

A Labrador and a poodle gives you a labradoodle. Floor and wardrobe create the mayhem of a floordrobe. Burqa plus bikini fashions a burkini.

Blends are the new black, from fusion cuisine to Googlegangers. (And don't pretend you haven't looked. Everybody does, which is why egosurfing is in the dictionary—another blend.)

So why should crossword clues be any different? If dog breeds can't keep their pedigree, then why must containers and reversals? Charades and homophones?

Whenever I'm encouraging wordy kids to try their luck at cryptic crosswords, I tend to sidestep the hybrid clue. Adult beginners get the same sympathy. The prospect of dealing with blended clues can prove overwhelming—a mongrel too wild to handle, despite the formulas being familiar in isolation.

By now, having reached this point in the book, you already know the nuts and bolts. You know how anagrams behave, how containers swaddle and spoonerisms spoonerise. A blended duet should be no scarier. All you need to do is identify each trick in succession, and the clue will crack.

It's more brainwork, true, but also more buzz when the answer arrives. Let's consider an example, if only to realise that a hybrid mongrel can be one cute labradoodle. This Arachne clue combines anagram and charade:

Fallen plumes arranged end to end (7)

Arranged should trigger a siren in your mind—a primary anagram indicator. *Plumes*, the abutting word, accounts for six letters, with one letter needed to reach the bracketed total of seven. What's that letter? And where does it come from?

End to end appears the likely phrase, a sly expression to imply the letter D, or the *end to end*. Attach that D onto rearranged *plumes*, and SLUMPE+D is your reward, or *fallen*.

Keeping with feathers, let's look at a Falcon clue from the *Financial Times*, this time the cocktail entailing deletion and anagram:

Follow dancing queens? Not initially (5)

Once again, the definition is embodied by the opening word, *follow*. Once more a common anagram signpost is planted in the clue's next segment, *dancing* this time. Yet before those *queens* kick up their heels, something needs removing, as suggested by the final deletion component: *Not initially*.

Lose the Q and dance with the remaining five—*ueens*. Do you follow all this? If you do, then endorphins ENSUE.

Congratulations. You have now reached the final bunch of example clues—ten this time, to encompass the breadth of hybrid combos (which I've identified in brackets beside each specimen). Cover those ingredients if you'd rather decode each clue as it comes.

Please don't agonise if you barely solve a handful of the ten—or none, for that matter. Only experience—untold hours of mental gymnastics—will turn these tigons (ferocious tiger–lion hybrids) into so many adorable kitties.

| E | X | A | M | P | L | E | S | | | | | | | | | |

Hybrid clues

1. *Shrewd like trustee, every now and then* (6) [Dac—charade/alternation]
2. *Aim always, say, to try hard* (9) [Rufus—charade/homophone]
3. *Lying bum flogged modern houses* (9) [Picaroon—anagram/container]
4. *Performed reflected melody with punch* (7) [Henry Hook—charade/reversal]
5. *Klutz upended flagon regularly* (3) [DA—alternation/reversal]
6. *Explain cryptic clue, I see* (9) [Puck—anagram/charade]
7. *Banks leaving Barbados to move overseas* (6) [Arachne—deletion/anagram]
8. *Working across part of garden without a pick* (6) [Anglio—container/deletion]
9. *Large within and without, turning smooth* (4) [Times 10,762—container/reversal]
10. *Village People's original backing hits now remastered* (8) [SK—charade/anagram]

ANSWERS: 1. AS+TUTE, **2.** END+EAVOUR, **3.** REC[UMB*]ENT, **4.** SANG+RIA<, **5.** OAF<, **6.** ELUC<I+DATE, **7.** ABROAD*, **8.** O[P/a/RTIO]N, **9.** G[LI]B<, **10.** TOWNSHI*+P

B O O S T E R ▮ P A C K

Top ten tips for solving success

Gym junkies know the rush that a workout brings. Yoga fans speak of feel-good chemicals flushing the system, loosening the knots that stress inflicts on the body. But maybe these last two chapters have had the opposite effect? Is your brain still giddy from the cryptic knots you've tried to loosen, a vague sense of panic growing in your stomach?

That's natural. Your neurons have been through a lot. After so many wordplay styles, a primer in punctuation and then a mess of hybrids, you're likely feeling concussed. Even if you managed to navigate the examples, solve your share, and learn a few traps, your cortex is bound to seem like Semtex, ready to explode.

Your working memory may well resemble something like a cyber-catalogue—a sketchy archive of signposts and recipes afloat in the medial lobe. Thus it will stay, fading over time, unless you return to the contest. Sure, you may be hip to rebuses right now, or have the knack to pinpoint a homophone, but will you twig to the same categories in a month? A year?

The answer is yes, so long as you practise, and practise, and practise a little more. That's what Part Three is for, your chance to convert the data into second nature. It sounds like drudgery, but not once that light floods your skull, the bliss of cracking your first clue in that first crossword.

Ask any solver: they all remember their first conquered clue, that triumph of a first completed grid. Solving begets solving, the aha pleasures never diminishing. And solving *improves* solving, the sketchy archive morphing into declarative memory, the long-term kind that etches a skill-set for life.

All that awaits you in the puzzles to come, both here in this book and beyond the covers. Before we leave this how-to section, however, here are a few tips for the road.

More hints than rules, a list to clear your path to solving success, the tips will ensure that next crossword will slowly unravel with the right amount of brainpower.

Give the list a read, and give it heed. There's no point in knowing the formulas only to be discouraged when first trying to spot them in the wild. Those tricks are coming in spades. But first, take time to save time.

1. **PICK THE RIGHT LEVEL.** Crosswords vary from quick to un-quick, from start-up puzzles with obvious deceits to the opaque hellhouse of British themers, the likes of *The Listener*'s barred diagrams that presume a working knowledge of Wagnerian maidens or pre-war exchequers. But most of all: be kind to yourself. Seek the puzzles that share their secrets at an encouraging rate, rewarding your solving at regular intervals. Don't expect your brain to recognise the tough stuff if you're only new to the genre. Find that happy place as a solver and evolve from there.

2. **SEEK OUT TWO-SPEED CLUES**, like the pair of puzzles that lie ahead. This is where two sets of clues—one quick, one cryptic—lead to the same set of answers. This style of puzzle is a major help, enabling your brain to switch from overt to covert language, giving you an insight as to where the definition sits in each cryptic clue. (As I write, an excellent example of this twin-clue format appears in *The Big Issue*—one more reason to buy the biweekly magazine that supports the disadvantaged.)

3. **CHEAT.** That's what I said—cheat. Peek at the answer if the clue seems impossible. At least that way you can work backwards, knowing that CHAMELEON is hiding in CLEAN HOME, since the lizard is the confirmed answer. And if this seems the low road to you, then call it reverse-engineering, a euphemism guaranteed to make you sleep more soundly. Besides, peeking proves you at least have the necessary curiosity, if not the willpower. Cheating, let's be honest, is a cocktail of teaching, and the more answers you swipe (fairly or grubbily), the quicker you'll expose the next clue's skulduggery.

4. **SHORT IS SWEET** in the realm of Cryptopia. Two-worded clues (with no question mark to suggest a pun) are almost always a double definition, such as '*Quality bore* (7)'. While the answer may not leap out, there should be some ease in knowing the particular formula you face. In this case, you know you seek a word that means quality, and one that means bore. How speedily you arrive at CALIBRE depends on your brainpower and your experience.

5. **1-ACROSS IS JUST A SUGGESTION.** In a perfect world, you'd solve 1-across, and then 1-down, and then 2-across and so on, the whole crossword collapsing like a house of cards. But as the hint above suggests, the shrewd solver will 'case the puzzle' before deciding where to break into the grid, sussing several clues to expose the easiest entry point.

6. **FIRST OR LAST**—that's the mantra to recite when parsing any clue. Because if most cryptic clues are made up of two parts—the wordplay and the definition, or vice versa—then it stands to reason that the answer's definition resides in either the clue's first word (or words), or the last. Try each extreme in turn, drumming up synonyms or possible responses to the word/s you find, and measure them against what the grid expects.

7. **PRIMING THE BRAIN** boosts your chances. Say you're tackling a puzzle's corner with one answer still to come. Don't just look at the corresponding clue cold. Instead, take a moment to consider what words might fit the pattern. If the cross-running letters give you C_R_E, then keep your feelers poised for any allusions to sculpture (CARVE), or radium (CURIE), or possibly an arc (CURVE). That way you'll be less likely to curse, should the clue seem bamboozling.

8. **OVERLOOK NOTHING**, including a clue's most inconspicuous word. Setters can't afford to add redundant language. Each word plays its part in a clue and no word is wasted. That's why it pays to read a clue aloud, slowly and methodically, knowing every word has a reason for being there. Now and then that word could link the two parts, or provide a finer detail to the definition, but the

rest can't afford to be skimmed. Each word is up to something. This includes words parading in one sense (squash—the drink, say) in the clue's surface meaning, only to mutate into squash the verb, or the veggie or perhaps the court game. In short: be suspicious. Words can be treacherous. If each clue is a gang of words, then every member's implicated.

9. **TAKE A WALK**. Make a cuppa. Get back to 'real' work. And by the time you resume the puzzle, your brain will deliver those solutions you couldn't reach in the first sitting. It happens every time, and the chapter 'Aha' tells us why. The knack depends on 'owning the problem' in the first place, giving the teaser enough think-time to register on the internal hard-drive. Take that vital break, and your gamma waves will lose their frenzy, allowing the eerie mode of subconscious thought to take sway—otherwise known as thinking when you don't seem to be thinking. An hour ago, let's say, you kept gazing at '*Spot of reckless drinking* (7)', failing to see beyond the clue's boozy picture. After taking a spell, feeding the goldfish and writing an email, your brain is now able to see *of reckless* plainly *drinking* FRECKLE, which is a *spot*, and your solution. That's the power of the so-called idle mind.

10. **FIND A FRIEND**, a lover, a workmate, a rellie. Sit down and solve with them. Side-by-side, the speculations will flow, for lots of reasons. Two brains are better than one, of course. But equally the rhythms of co-solving are ideal for isolating a clue's language—often by reciting the clues between each other, which converts the clues to audio, a mode better suited to free association. Even better, read the clue very slowly and deliberately, *word by word*. Make the language an identity parade, where the suspect term steps forward. Finally, deny it all you like, but solving as a duo will also elicit the age-old spur of competition, lending each eureka bonus kudos.

AND HAVE FUN, if I can add Tip 11, though that's akin to telling a horse to drink. Cryptic clues aim to frustrate and elate in equal measure. Their mission is to mislead, while your mission is to look past the lie, and thereby see where the answer's lying. That's the game of it. False trails are part of the treasure hunt. Even the sharpest solvers are fooled, which only goes to deepen the rush once the right trail is found.

Hence you want a puzzle that misleads just the right amount, to paraphrase Goldilocks. Too easy and you'll fill the grid in a trance. Too hard and the ahas will evaporate. But find the right level of evasiveness, and the pleasures are guaranteed.

Fingers crossed, you find that pleasure lurking in the puzzles to come, where every degree of difficulty awaits, from the garden variety to the OMG. I suggest you sharpen those wits and pencils and pounce on the final collection at leisure. Trust me: your brain will thank you.

PART THREE

THE

WT F

Fifty puzzles to keep your brain abuzz

The bending begins

The next 50 puzzles promise to deliver the wow and the wonder of cryptic clues, as well as the head-spin that comes with tackling such teasers.

We open with a series of six samplers—Formula foretastes—where each mini-puzzle displays its wordplay formula, from anagram to homophone. The approach is designed for familiarity, to get your brain accustomed to the shape and feel of each style, establishing a set of patterns that will slowly permeate your explicit memory.

From there we move to blended puzzles in a series called Recipes revealed, where each clue's operation is declared in ensuing brackets. This will spare the tyro's brain from pursuing false trails, as soon that folly will be all yours to enjoy.

Survive those six, resorting to the recipe notes if necessary, and you'll encounter a further half a dozen, labelled Recipes on request. For this series, each clue's formula is disclosed below each set of clues. In other words, the urge to peek gets a little less incidental, entailing a conscious decision to seek a friendly nudge if every other avenue has been pursued. Consider this bracket of puzzles—with recipes a glance away—as the nearest thing to solving solo.

That feat is fast approaching. Part Three is dedicated to letting you loose in Cryptopia, but not before one more important detour, visiting a pair of two-speed crosswords. Here two sets of clues—one quick, one cryptic—lead to the same solutions. Again, consult the quick clues only if you need guidance, your chance to confirm where the definition sits within each cryptic clue. Otherwise, if you're feeling game, ignore the quick clues wholesale, and treat each Two-speed challenge as one-speed only.

After that, beyond these warm-up puzzles, lies a 30-puzzle sequence of lobe-stretching crosswords, with no revelations aside from those your own brain generates. To smooth the way, I've arranged this final series according to difficulty, presenting three levels: Friendly (a relative term), Tricky and Gnarly. After that, to test your cerebrum to the max, you have a handful of themed puzzles as the last hurrah. Or aha.

Down the back, to ensure your future eurekas multiply, you'll find the answers are accompanied by brief notes, letting you see how the different ruses operate, from reversal to manipulation. Sharpen the wits, the pencils, and happy grappling.

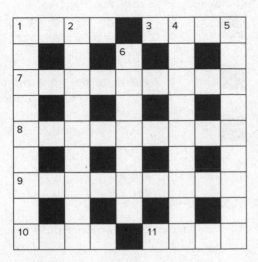

Puzzle 1 Formula foretaste I—Anagram

Hint: Look for the signpost in each clue, that signal to skew adjacent letters.

ACROSS
1. Harry, Ned—a boy's name (4)
3. So shut off (4)
7. I peter out, spoiling spin (9)
8. It decreases Mortein, as sprayed? (5,4)
9. Stir their mash, needing more water (9)
10. Enid arranged feast (4)
11. Spent fraudulent dues (4)

DOWN
1. Edits OpEd, roughly put in (9)
2. 1-across neighbour wearing no threads (9)
4. Most Irish plays haphazard (3-2-4)
5. Greenside Complex erupting (6,3)
6. Guess turned mussier (7)

Puzzle 2   Formula foretaste II—Hidden

Hint: Each clue hides its solution in plain sight.

ACROSS

4   French writer contributes to Gitmo lie readily (7)

5   Stupid basin in empty passage (7)

6   China's potential partly stuck (2,1,4)

DOWN

1   Agree to lexicon's entire excerpt (7)

2   'Big cat' in Swahili, one's supposing (7)

3   Club ran so noisily, stuffing entrepreneur (7)

Puzzle 3   Formula foretaste III—Double definition

Hint: No signposts are required in this formula, where two definitions for the one solution sit hand-in-hand.

ACROSS

3   Contemporary ocean motion (7)

5   Warmer Princess Di, once upon a time? (7)

6   Decreed in sequence (7)

DOWN

1   Field athletes' guernseys (7)

2   Catalogued like a hand? (7)

4   Stove set (5)

Puzzle 4   Formula foretaste IV—Charade

Hint: NUMBAT is NUMB plus AT in this habitat, no scrambling needed. That's why charades lack signposts, although they may carry their share of linking words. You'll find this puzzle the hardest so far.

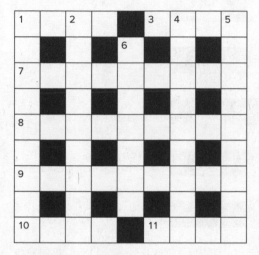

ACROSS

  1   Rate parliament's foremost expert (4)
  3   English male needs mother to get Austen novel (4)
  7   Withdrew on pay for singer Sheeran (9)
  8   Shop's interior making meal, plus one movie (4,5)
  9   Awful eastern golfer, Norman, acquired debts (9)
 10   Brownish potassium vat (4)
 11   Gather the girl's diamonds (4)

DOWN

  1   Ancient paper published first by crafty men on time (9)
  2   Whip a blemish on a new twin-hulled boat (9)
  4   Timekeeper met director Howard to ring me (9)
  5   Dealt with a daughter in clothing (9)
  6   Muddle me with NZ's ex-PM, David (7)

Puzzle 5   Formula foretaste V—Container

Hint: MACRAME can be RAM surrounded by MACE, or MACE swamping RAM—or even A CRAM squashing into ME. Because in this recipe, X holds Y, or Y disrupts X.

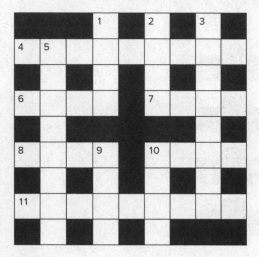

ACROSS

4   Height gauge to change across duration (9)
6   Expert covered nephew's first zits (4)
7   Crazy to hug one servant (4)
8   Bump torpedo's head aboard *Nautilus*? (4)
10   Bloke interrupts morning: 'Excuse me!' (4)
11   Napoleon has a role, cutting fillet (9)

DOWN

1   Fib about new wrinkle (4)
2   Masterpiece infected by radical microbe (4)
3   US money injected into broadcast dregs (8)
5   Place to find calcium-laced cream? (8)
9   Craft Club hemming zip? (4)
10   US city, as circumscribed sadly (4)

Puzzle 6   Formula foretaste VI—Homophone

Hint: While homophone clues are easy to 'sea', thanks to their audio cue, they do call on two steps: find the wordplay's word, then say that word aloud. (Beware: one clue entails a double homophone, where two words need vocalising to sound out the solution.)

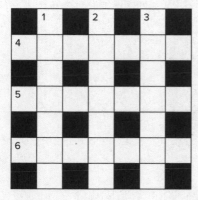

ACROSS

4 Painter's need a sense of taste, we hear (7)
5 Impressive AFL marks aircraft sheds, say (7)
6 Audited fringe lodger (7)

DOWN

1 Bullfighter issue opening under discussion? (7)
2 Report shelves account books (7)
3 Levels quoted in accounts (7)

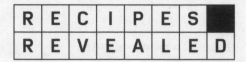

Puzzle 7 Recipes revealed I

For the next six puzzles, you have the advantage of knowing which formula each clue uses. But even knowing that, will you intuit the answer?

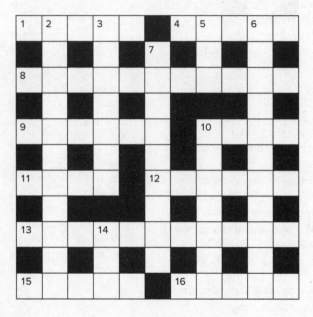

ACROSS

1   Notices measles (5) [double definition]
4   Prevents 1-across spreading (5) [anagram]
8   Accountant to head bench (4-7) [charade]
9   Choice meat to satisfy alien (6) [charade]
10   Turn tots around (4) [reversal]
11   Briefly learn poker variety (4) [deletion]
12   Cold stretch extending police capacity? (6) [hidden]
13   Cocktail jumper (11) [double definition]
15   Derelict acre's cow (5) [anagram]
16   So-called snake box (5) [homophone]

DOWN

2   Hip rector is surprisingly old (11) [anagram]
3   Taste guided Rapunzel movie (7) [charade]
5   Oddly tie in X (3) [alternation]
6   Fix absolutely divine clothing (11) [container]
7   Loudly battled 14-down for two weeks (9) [homophone x 2]
10   Overnight carriage for dark horse? (7) [double definition]
14   Galahad perhaps smiles into romantic faces (3) [code]

Puzzle 8 Recipes revealed II

A hybrid clue is lurking in this one. Will you have the combo mojo?

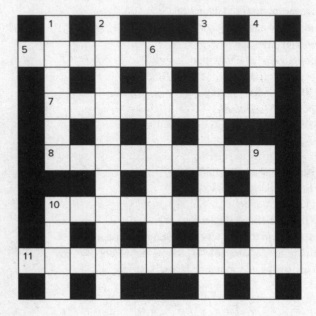

ACROSS

5 Small cart section on 'Jolene' singer (5,6) [charade]

7 Terrible pill abuse can be believed (9) [anagram]

8 Discovered Dante caters for echidnas? (9) [deletion]

10 Picked up, bored with cows, say? (9) [charade/homophone]

11 Maori cousin turned bitter (11) [anagram]

DOWN

1 Fuss is fair game (4-2) [double definition]

2 Dispel tensions at rare Chile conflict (5,3,3) [anagram]

3 Awkward butcher to price lamb (11) [anagram]

4 One individual on radio (4) [homophone]

6 Nut, oats, chip I crunch (9) [anagram]

9 Element of skinhead hatred (6) [charade]

10 Top fell off sofa—that hurt! (4) [deletion]

Puzzle 9 Recipes revealed III

What—no anagram?! Tough, but you should thrive.

ACROSS

1 Quoted trim couple (4) [homophone]
4 Thai region as Opiate Central? (4) [charade]
7 Touch wicked to retreat (3) [reversal]
9 Grub to feed Parthenon supporter? (11) [charade]
10 Dad's stabbing some odd jerk (5) [container/alternation]
11 Old language elating insiders (5) [hidden]
12 Triumphant cry, even on reflection (3) [reversal]
13 Initially terse, small-time message? (5) [charade]
14 Record raised funds (5) [homophone]
16 CO144ME? (5,6) [rebus]
18 Name kids' game (3) [double definition]
19 Increased writing, head down (4) [deletion]
20 Initial bloke to reject crazy airhead (4) [reversal]

DOWN

1 Gently kisses chest muscles, say (5) [homophone]
2 Quaint raven ousted screens of an ER tube? (11) [hidden]
3 Exploit dance style (3) [double definition]
5 Go back twinkling (5,6) [double definition x 2]
6 For an outer kitchen garment (5) [container]
7 Beckett maybe shot at first (9) [charade]
8 Charge a water pipe connecting waterhole (9) [charade]
13 Cat steps with agility, leaving ground in seconds (5) [code]
15 Imagine weir swamping 19-across's tips (5) [container]
17 I get article on novelist Rankin (3) [charade]

Puzzle 10 Recipes revealed IV

Classically, when Cockneys head for home, they 'ead for 'ome. That 'abit will 'elp you with 5-down.

ACROSS

1   Excel to hold up bakery? (4,3,4) [pun]
7   Dug retro material (5) [reversal]
8   Ratbag and French apprentice (5) [charade]
9   It protects bar's pet straying behind the clock (11) [anagram/charade]
11 Relics sit in quite a mess (11) [anagram]
12 Called one to cover Greek character? (5) [homophone]
14 Beethoven's last symphony began in the series (5) [hidden]
16 Web-handlers mishandling Euro kingdom (11) [charade/anagram]

DOWN

1   Small portion cheers Democrat (3) [charade]
2   Gentlest family destined to lose half (7) [charade/deletion]
3   NYC's own X^2? (5,6) [rebus]
4   Special translation of a pet lexicon (11) [anagram]
5   Cockney assistant, a joiner? (3) [deletion]
6   Skipping starts, gent frees starters (7) [deletion]
9   Beck ran feral in fernery (7) [anagram]
10 Idiot travelled north, after touring via French city (7) [reversal/anagram]
13 Stone quarry (3) [double definition]
15 Gets laughter? (3) [double definition]

Puzzle 11   Recipes revealed V

A bit of bilingualism required in this puzzle. *Bon chance!*

ACROSS

1   Flier injured arm (5) [anagram]
4   Painter Pablo 'so' ditching print measures (5) [deletion]
7   Ponder prisoner attending church at breaks (11) [charade/container]
8   Outstanding pair in Rome (3) [double definition—one in Italian!]
9   A mate might start radar, perhaps (7) [charade]
10 Some cold wind levels slide (7) [hidden]
11 Sort of dog circuit? (3) [double definition]
13 Vulnerable one gives session nothing (7,4) [charade]
14 Wander right into stop (5) [container]
15 Snobs kept off space capsule (5) [hidden]

DOWN

1   Guillotine found bolted (5) [deletion]
2   Spooner to sense fitter as indecisive person (5-6) [spoonerism]
3   Melt a dry-ice mixture in Oz destination (7,4) [anagram]
4   Quiet mimic heard to hang around desk item (11) [charade/homophone]
5   Ride the remote waterway waves? (7-4) [pun]
6   Send the electricity across, matching leads for power source (5) [code]
10 Deer swallow small intakes (5) [container]
12 Keeps wild dogs (5) [anagram]

Puzzle 12   Recipes revealed VI

What series is complete without a themed puzzle? And a *scary* one to boot. This is your toughest challenge to date, so be kind to yourself.

ACROSS

1 Custom to decline during cure, occasionally (5) [container/alternation]
4 Fleet satirist (5) [double definition]
8 Backstage may rate lousy 2-down creation (3,8) [reversal/anagram]
9 Goes outside, seizing 10-across for spirits (6) [container]
10 Multitude run the show (4) [double definition]
11 Catch horses, tail-first (4) [manipulation]
13 Killer US poet Walt starting off (6) [deletion]
15 Tired star is rejoining UK band (4,7) [anagram]
16 Spy needs years to reach central frontier (5) [charade]
17 Bear to mention 2-down novel (5) [homophone]

DOWN

2 Writer presents layer after layer to sovereign (7,4) [charade]
3 2-down's readers' responses perhaps linking back to snakes (5) [charade]
5 Vigil needing ticker? (5) [pun]
6 Kinky trait refers to 2-down's book (11) [anagram]
7 Cryptically this arises, like many of 2-down's books (5,4) [partial rebus]
12 Information about lines describing 2-down's mile (5) [container]
14 Partly graffiti Arabic crown (5) [hidden]

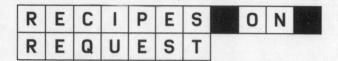

Puzzle 13   Recipes on request I

Time to unhitch the safety net. Feel free to peek at the 'Recipes on request' box below each set of clues for any clue's formula in the next six puzzles. But test your nerves—and nous—before you do.

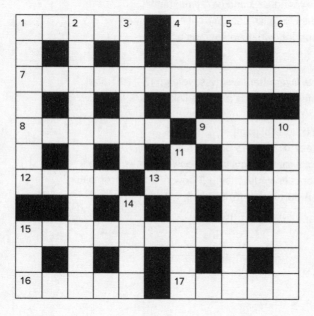

ACROSS

1   Card-game jabber? (5)
4   Cyclist clipped big kerb (5)
7   A man won heart by extent of defoliant (5,6)
8   Must split before small rebellion (6)
9   Token golf shot (4)
12   Total love for Japanese wrestling (4)
13   Live-in nanny suggests gold earrings? (2,4)
15   Vital finance for Astle start-up of the brain? (11)
16   Heard to gather in West Africa (5)
17   Did boy cut oxygen supply to old lady? (5)

DOWN

1   Actor Neill's peak-climbing on TVs? (7)
2   Condition where you need to take something? (11)
3   Eye part of turret in Alhambra precinct (6)
4   Sent up boring poet (4)
5   Warm, heated drink spilt (4-7)
6   Paddle in sound for fish eggs (3)
10   Leaves players reeling? (7)
11   Singly pierced U-boat? Brilliant! (6)
14   War dance that makes shaky guts (4)
15   Travel north after forest's initial driving hazard (3)

Puzzle 14 Recipes on request II

Three cheers if you solve 11-across without peeking. Easily the hardest clue in the grid.

ACROSS

1 Observed mail price fluctuating (9)
8 Tricky topic of eyes (5)
9 Hindi area essentially! (5)
10 Empty promise of upper crust? (3,2,3,3)
11 Figure outlines curve in joint inflammation (6,5)
14 Skimmed firm diagram (5)
15 Names for 'semesters'? (5)
16 Fruit crate repacked to fill square (9)

DOWN

2 Dull substance reduced (5)
3 Prone to going, visiting Africa maybe? (11)
4 Flower originally held for me and dog? (5,6)
5 Range across Arabian Desert (5)
6 Tricky topic creating wedge? (3,6)
7 Rap star turning wet and sneaky (5,4)
12 Thanklessly notable 13-down, perhaps (5)
13 Eavesdropped unproductive court figure (5)

Recipes on request II

ACROSS:

1 anagram
8 anagram
9 hidden &lit
10 pun
11 charade/anagram/charade
14 deletion
15 double definition
16 anagram/container

DOWN:

2 deletion
3 charade
4 charade
5 hidden
6 pun
7 anagram
12 deletion
13 homophone

Puzzle 15   Recipes on request III

Spoonerism, code, homophone, &lit—there's a full rollcall of recipes in this grid. But which clue obeys which formula?

ACROSS

1 Boundlessly harsh way back for London XI (7)
7 Each aunt I'll organise to see things (11)
8 Free ladies sent off base? (6)
9 Tropical getaway regularly insulted (4)
11 Report: 'Look for bloke in turban' (4)
12 Releases Spooner's ducks? (4,2)
14 Tolkien's setting art, cryptically (6-5)
15 Sketch harbour fish (7)

DOWN

1 Anxious Pearl would somehow bandage kid's head (3,6,2)
2 Drunk thoroughly exploited (6)
3 New city written up in detective fiction (4)
4 Deceives protagonists botching art, say (5,6)
5 Short ladies keep spaces pure (9)
6 Monsters demolished Beth's home (9)
10 Fragment—remote?! (6)
13 Starts to suffer loneliness under racial insult (4)

Recipes on request III

ACROSS		DOWN	
1	deletion/reversal	1	anagram/container
7	anagram	2	charade
8	charade/deletion	3	reversal/charade
9	alternation	4	charade/anagram
11	homophone	5	deletion/container
12	spoonerism	6	anagram
14	rebus	10	anagram &lit
15	charade	13	code

Puzzle 16   Recipes on request IV

If setters are allowed to pick a favourite within a puzzle series, then here's mine. Put your brain in 15-down.

ACROSS

1 No more shooting boater, possibly cut in snare (5,1,4)
8 Strike put out field event (6,5)
9 Current event arranged online (2,4)
10 Slight rolls to the west (4)
12 Dressing might demo bottom (4)
14 Fellow gets licence to kill penguin (6)
17 Summer Ale so intoxicated dashing chap? (6,5)
18 Gathering habit (10)

DOWN

2 Rambo romantic at heart when on edge (2-3)
3 Kicking drawing, say (6)
4 Bohemian bash going topless (4)
5 Repeated lecturer and nurses (5)
6 He lends money to Spooner's card-game with muscle (10)
7 Slyly use chemist notepaper? (5,5)
11 Frog-kick initially okay after head sagged (6)
13 Red Sea nation blasted enemy (5)
15 High-powered duck getting dry when moving north (5)
16 I duplicated viral video (4)

Recipes on request IV

ACROSS
1 charade/container
8 charade
9 anagram
10 reversal
12 charade
14 charade
17 anagram
18 double definition

DOWN
2 charade
3 homophone
4 deletion
5 hidden
6 spoonerism
7 anagram
11 charade/deletion
13 anagram
15 reversal/charade
16 charade

Puzzle 17   Recipes on request V

Commonly in Cryptopia, 'I' denotes 'me', or vice versa. Though across my puzzles, when I say 'I' that could signify DA, my puzzle-page by-line. PS: 4-down is tough.

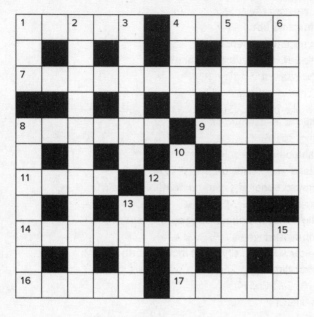

ACROSS

1 I get paunch—that's a fact (5)
4 Loquacious pig added to large hubbub (5)
7 Flip logical bits out (2,9)
8 Humdrum bum occupies vacuous day (6)
9 Meat full of vitamins? (4)
11 Commentator's spots to stretch (4)
12 Chest of audible flu sufferer maybe (6)
14 Expecting sign isn't, for example (11)
16 Female 17-across in retiring . . . (5)
17 . . . advantage, like planned (5)

DOWN

1 Enjoyed drudge, oddly (3)
2 Pill-mixing insane—abandoning a sport? (5,6)
3 Grinder's second Swede? (6)
4 Dash upset writer's innards (4)
5 Queasy feeling is close to numb, say—quickly passes (11)
6 Devil cruel if provoked (7)
8 Tonally deaf—is it shortfall? (7)
10 Caught stabbing gloomy rocker with a prankster's cry (6)
13 Giant peddler in East End (4)
15 Macadamia maniac (3)

Recipes on request V

ACROSS

1 charade
4 charade
7 anagram
8 container
9 charade
11 homophone
12 homophone
14 double definition
16 reversal
17 charade

DOWN

1 alternation
2 charade/anagram/deletion
3 charade
4 manipulation
5 charade
6 anagram
8 homophone
10 container/charade
13 homophone
15 double definition

Puzzle 18   Recipes on request VI

There's a reason this one wraps the series. In a word: ouch. But remember, if pain persists, every recipe is in easy reach.

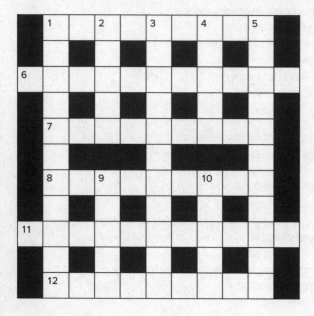

ACROSS

1 Indulged, rested lives, given food around one (9)
6 UK pal possibly scoffing ex-PM (4,7)
7 Sit still, editing video's end on TV mode (2,3,4)
8 Fuel-coated skirts made womanly (9)
11 Ex-PM found with pot and shades, we hear (5,6)
12 He'd assert changes for dental chairs' features (9)

DOWN

1 Aloof trawlerman's stall? (11)
2 Hair boutique putting aside capital for true gripper? (5)
3 It slows a ship down to pick up woman on ship (5,6)
4 Start distributing rations as evacuating (5)
5 Sir ends imbroglio, clothing dweeb in formal wear (6,5)
9 Mum orbited key island (5)
10 Traces trigonometric curves in auditorium (5)

Recipes on request VI

ACROSS
1 charade/container
6 anagram/charade
7 anagram
8 container
11 charade/homophone
12 anagram

DOWN
1 charade
2 manipulation
3 homophone x 2
4 deletion/anagram
5 anagram/container
9 container
10 homophone

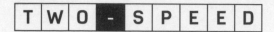

Puzzle 19 Two-speed crossword I—General

Quick clues like 15-down—*Make*—can only make.trouble, since that word owns a raft of synonyms, from build to earn to model and so on. Most candidates, however, will vanish when you consider the corresponding cryptic clue for the same solution. Choose whichever clue-speed you'd rather, but keep in mind the cryptic style gives you two glimpses of the answer, if you know where to look.

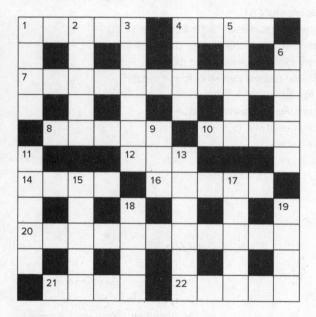

CRYPTIC CLUES

ACROSS

1 Season puts out new shoot (5)
4 Declared good time to cry (4)
7 Declaring policing arm corrupt (11)
8 Cook heads for some additive, usually to enrich (5)
10 Avoid blazer with hot lining? (4)
12 Sort of skimmed dairy product (3)

14 Arrive at the final part of brain (4)
16 Ellis wove cloth (5)
20 Charming Maria hits tremor in staccato midsection? (11)
21 Cheese produced in recession (4)
22 Briefly SMS an American (5)

DOWN

1   Exhausts nincompoops (4)
2   Girl distributing hoard (5)
3   Large Latin lodgers iced treats (6)
4   Bond to leave in a hurry (4)
5   Reported means to put on a scale (5)
6   Pain once nasty in flanks (5)
9   Some 115 cm evenly across sea-lily (3)
11 Pull out grit (5)
13 Devastating mistake, overlooking a fortune (6)
15 Mark grain on tapered end (5)
17 It gives delayed kiss (5)
18 Business movie switched sides (4)
19 Check disheartened Scotsman (4)

QUICK CLUES

ACROSS

1   Green shoot (5)
4   Yell (4)
7   Attesting (11)
8   Lightly fry (5)
10 Avoid (4)
12 Sort (3)
14 Brain segment (4)
16 Cotton fabric (5)
20 Exuding allure (11)
21 Dutch cheese (4)
22 Dallas local (5)

DOWN

1   Fools (4)
2   Unfashionable name for a girl (5)
3   Frozen treats (6)
4   Scoop (4)
5   Assess (5)
6   Pain (5)
9   Printing measure (3)
11 Courage (5)
13 Destiny (6)
15 Make (5)
17 Synthetic material (5)
18 Stable (4)
19 Read (4)

Puzzle 20 Two-speed crossword II—Bird word

This puzzle proves that 'quick' crosswords aren't. As per the last challenge, you face two sets of clues, leading to the one 'flock' of answers.

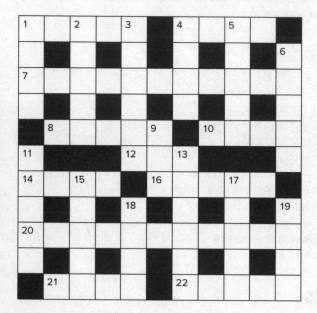

CRYPTIC CLUES

ACROSS

1 Unusual bumpkin holds record (5)
4 Worm's tip fulfilled darn sea duck (4)
7 Seabird tormented smelter port (5,6)
8 Heard small bird (5)
10 Check stalk (4)
12 Delay prisoner (3)
14 Warren dropped a river bird (4)
16 Dream up what can stop school threat in seconds (5)
20 Bird nearby can squall (11)
21 Seabird to spin on the air (4)
22 Online message gets dainty with time (5)

DOWN

1 Capone's mob stripped as well (4)
2 Scary cry by seabird (5)
3 Camel for one gets timid heart seeing camel heading off, we hear (6)
4 Bird food creates speed, not power (4)
5 Bit of detergent over bird (5)
6 Feather is magnificent on magpie's tail (5)
9 Heath oddly gives triumphant cry (3)
11 Sydney's AFL players faint for nothing during SOS (5)
13 Ten fuss about seabird (6)
15 Bird of prey decapitated dog (5)
17 Wading bird cocked head near ground (5)
18 Floor swept, unclean in the extreme (4)
19 Sent off bird shelter (4)

QUICK CLUES

ACROSS

1 Record (5)
4 Diving bird (4)
7 Seabird (5,6)
8 Asian bird (5)
10 Stop (4)
12 Trail (3)
14 Songbird (4)
16 Emerge, as a bird (5)
20 Songbird (11)
21 Seabird (4)
22 Bird-like utterance (5)

DOWN

1 Plus (4)
2 Seabird (5)
3 Cat, say—but not a catbird (6)
4 Bird food, often (4)
5 Wading bird (5)
6 Bird feature (5)
9 Derisive laugh (3)
11 Waterbirds (5)
13 Seabird (6)
15 Bird of prey (5)
17 Wading bird (5)
18 Wow (4)
19 Bird's home (4)

FRIENDLY CRYPTICS

Puzzle 21 Friendly I

No more handrails, or two-faced birds: our next series includes eight cryptic crosswords, minus recipe hints. But let's start slow, increasing the brain-load as we go.

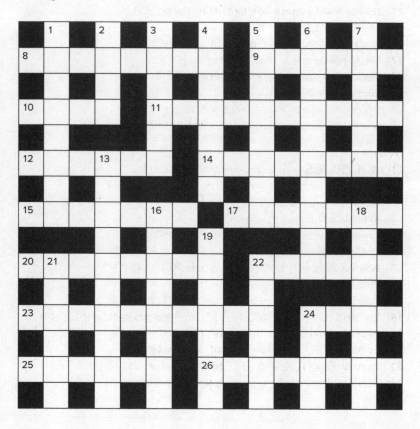

ACROSS

8   Hitches northward, OK (6-2)
9   You finally renovated patio—it's perfect! (6)
10 Piano number enshrines fertile writer? (4)
11 A derelict's eccentric liquid measures (10)
12 Bee's knees barely found in old Greek city (6)
14 Stressed doctors diagnose (8)
15,17-across,24-across   Yokel, or youth leader, gets detective, or youth leader, to cut nursery rhyme (7,7,4)
17 See 15-across
20 Revised, 4-down is loveless way to stand sailing (8)
22 Honest guide (6)
23 Military offsider developed idea to flee (4-2-4)
24 See 15-across
25 Mountain retreats take in Venus or Mars (6)
26 Sneak sleep inside, near a Sydney funfair (4,4)

DOWN

1   Wrongfully employ scissors—hang hair clump (8)
2   Zen chant reaching an Arabic nation (4)
3   Hit songs' digressions? (6)
4   Exceptional places I travelled (7)
5   Cryptic clue: 'Lion gets cellular bodies' (8)
6   Toady let go hard stuff for auditors (10)
7   Acquire 20 quires, say, for ancient galley (6)
13 Plain dish lambasted naked babes (5,5)
16 Casino game allowed to obstruct path (8)
18 It's often controversial to play this Flemington program, perhaps (4,4)
19 Warm Aesop story a female covers (7)
21 Alpine hanger-on discovered BMX, we hear (6)
22 Bank on dole? People need limits! (6)
24 Fool extremely dense to drink up (4)

Puzzle 22   Friendly II

Even if an answer is new to your vocab (such as 13-across, or 24-across, perhaps), a cryptic clue lends you a fighting chance via its wordplay.

ACROSS

1 Start to saw logs?! (7)
5 Bad omen upset stomach (7)
10 Small business got untidy crates repaired (7,8)
11 Wrong to pinch back-end of monkey? (6)
12 Spinning or cutting (8)
13 Residence prepared single divorce document (6,4)
15 Clean either side of willow tree (4)
17 Party buffet (4)
19 Pacific crop raised in sound, suitable to retain syrupy centre (10)
21 *Amoebae A-To-Z*, poor edition (8)
23 Cheers strike on one Pacific island (6)
24 Iraqi elite concerning taverner facing a drug bust (10,5)
25 Press heavies abuse steroid (7)
26 Prizes reflected athletics meet, serving hosts (7)

DOWN

2 The French ring number of king? (7)
3 Leading female Rita struggled during rally (9)
4 Spur description of a shamed face? (3,2)
6 Pump iron buddy! Boil bananas! (4-5)
7 Opening response that's withholding (5)
8 Casualty receives money for South African jobs (7)
9 Phone-in tactic deployed sticker to restrict drawing? (8,5)
13 Call knight (3)
14 Fraudster to breeze around with laundered money—zillions initially (9)
15 Wasted wee hours sealing a storage space (9)
16 Saucy, naked photo (3)
18 Bimbo to help flightless bird nesting (7)
20 Meanwhile, winter imperilled hostage (7)
22 Ridicule Dad's sister with tank-top (5)
23 Deliberately loses scuba gear (5)

Puzzle 23   Friendly III

1-across is no doddle, so don't bust the brain for too long. Move around instead.
Find the kinder clues and enter the grid that way.

ACROSS

1   Sets off charges to protect disc (7)
5   Place for acting surgeon? (7)
9   And not chew on the ear (3)
10 Factory needs years on web to produce royal French line (11)
11 Contrarily hides sheltered place for Soviet satellites (8)
12 Selected sides for coach—one's unpredictable (6)
15 Snowman in yard certain to melt oddly? (4)
16 White House translated Bogart–Bergman classic (10)
18 Detective to grunt and flirt? (7,3)
19 Arab leader quiet before aftermath ends (4)
22 Doctors' helpers squashed grapes (6)
23 Arrangement of pearl with one red gem (4,4)
25 Issues T-bone during Butcher Studies (11)
27 Pinch little drink (3)
28 He loved wrapping feral ostrich (7)
29 Robbery ringleader cuts into livestock grant (3,4)

DOWN

1   Heartless duty perverted 10-across, for one (7)
2   Spinning rake in olive process (11)
3   Again confined regret? (6)
4   Scramble and streak, exhibiting sleek bottom like this? (5,5)
5   Matching pair said to be tailor-made for 2-down? (4)
6   Yellowy-white barracks he'll join (8)
7   Fairly small preserve (3)
8   Splash in sea to land (7)
13 Don's sidekick devious on chap's stated solution (6,5)
14 She minds minibar next to studio model (4-6)
17 Famed tenor Jose gets $100 to tackle arrears (8)
18 Haitian dictator owns a flat, cased by detective from Down Under (4,3)
20 CEO maintains edge in landing spot (7)
21 Perhaps F-11s, with radio band, dumped stuff (6)
24 Spanish river partly absorbed ebbing (4)
26 Gentleman curtailed iPhone voice (3)

Puzzle 24   Friendly IV

Geography and Hollywood. Zoology and ball-sports. A cryptic square for the trivia all-rounder.

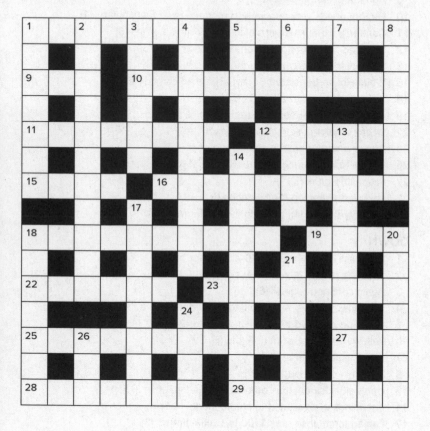

ACROSS

1   Some rhymes far from riveting? (7)
5   Rhythmic sound is bread-and-butter? (7)
9   Managed screen display (3)
10 Thought elder baited vagrant (11)
11 Get around foul tank spill (8)
12 Cloak upon chook section (6)
15 Possibly saw plunder going west (4)
16 Boor heard to serve at 25-across? (10)
18 Fluid study in daily crush, perhaps (10)
19 Sketch halved ninepins (4)
22 Wreck in a dock (6)
23 Sergeant shot blank (8)
25 Fine to be loud during remainder of grog-a-thon (11)
27 I improve golf slice (3)
28 Sprite exchanges $1000 at Russian castle (7)
29 Inadequate show to steer contradictory truth (7)

DOWN

1   Last offer (4,3)
2   Customised dream somehow buggered up inside (4-2-5)
3   Initially altered wee enigma (6)
4   Sound dog carries fruit down (10)
5   Bars turn up bands? (4)
6   Wrong racket uncovered amphibian (8)
7   Sink vessel (3)
8   Little frog bit European (7)
13 Coop grain or peanuts? (7,4)
14 Rocky Beach's kelp outcast (5,5)
17 Can writer supervise a large man-eater? (8)
18 Noah's son on faux-bed (7)
20 Actor Justin—protagonist in formal attire? (7)
21 Packer seen on the moon? (6)
24 DA 9-across country (4)
26 Little piggy to leave behind? (3)

Puzzle 25 Friendly V

All four longer entries involve anagrams in some way. Hence the friendly rating, but will you crack the puzzle in toto?

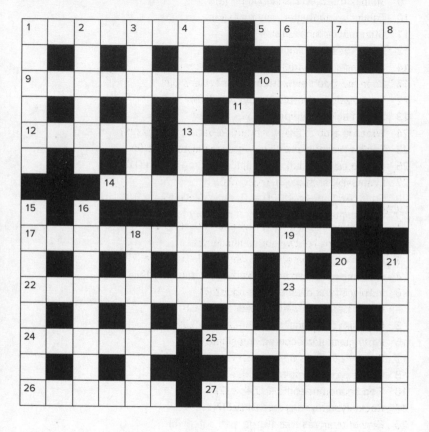

ACROSS

1   Pluck tree-top in wind (8)
5   Avoid Dutch illusionist dropping his last showstopper (6)
9   Shapes to 26-across speakers? (8)
10 Calumnies implicated graduates (6)
12 Utter power impairs (5)
13 Willing bear and eagle to tussle (9)
14 Composer can harm break by pool error (12)
17 Supreme Court exploited mouse owner? (8,4)
22 French father accepts cut to keep going (9)
23 Same backlot tidier in part (5)
24 Supplies grub to Blanchett and Roberts on fringes (6)
25 Terribly nice rug sporting a Picasso masterpiece (8)
26 Calm male pursuing smut (6)
27 Eventually tenth gal changed (2,6)

DOWN

1   Aussie parrots loiter over scattered ash (6)
2   Shop detains lightweight composer (6)
3   Crack unit eliminated continent's leader in Africa (7)
4   I revere havoc becoming extravagant success (12)
6   2-down's rival dressed falsehood? (7)
7   Heard that bloke reserve church tome (8)
8   Demolish immediately on the phone (5,3)
11 Party game somehow nurtures hate (8,4)
15 Preserve choices for mountaineering gear (3-5)
16 A horse to swallow tiptop liqueur (8)
18 Find caribou near the squirrels (7)
19 Cockney's slow galloper, okay? (7)
20 Kind of quartet series (6)
21 Field hospital included on Melbourne campus (6)

Puzzle 26   Friendly VI

Reverend Spooner makes his Part Three debut. He's simple to spot, compared to a sneakier code clue that's also implicated.

ACROSS

1 Confectionery to stuff final cost (6)
4 Bloody irate charity (3,5)
9 Slacker times integral to genuine retirement (5)
10 Venetian and I trashed Laos capital (9)
11 Return embargo on bundle (9)
12 Provide online gag? (5)
13 Qualification (with hesitations) for personal trainers? (12)
17 Old redhead is tribe's only rebel (5,7)
20 Cockney paradises for Oz cycle champ (5)
21 Max needs a nap or stretch to find peace, historically (3,6)
23 Clubs revised up-to-date power grab (4,1'4)
24 Banned bill on ducks? (5)
25 Catastrophe as anticyclone enclosed game (8)
26 He fishes for laptop amid fury (6)

DOWN

1 Radio format to be fresh? (8)
2 Spooner's pawns established dog breed (8)
3 Spectre's close to Lake Strange (5)
5 My energetic ex undid escape hatch (9,4)
6 Church pet shredded *Herald* (9)
7 Pop a question, somewhat dense (6)
8 Plain pace recorded (6)
10 17-across's successor contested valid margin reverting to Labour? (8,5)
14 Cromwellians throwing derisions (9)
15 Is brown bovine docked in Turkey? (8)
16 Liked four vain models (2,6)
18 Vessel stops near Pacific Ocean, bursts open in seconds (6)
19 Do for a gardener? (6)
22 Frequently decimal? (5)

Puzzle 27 Friendly VII

16-down is perhaps your toughest clue so far, followed closely by 14-down. Meaning the grid's south-east corner presents a real showdown.

ACROSS

7   Unbridled energy is very, very cool (8)
9   Chuck visits Zoroastrian's ultimate paradise (6)
10   Articulate chief reduced weight (4)
11   Sydney race cuts tyro, if staggering (4,2,4)
12   Clear soup hardly commonest variety (8)
14   Hangs physician? That's a mistake! (6)
15   Abandoned isle we chose (OK?) for October hijinks (9,4)
17   Impoverished duo minimised stringed instrument in wings (4-2)
19   Work (Sawyer novel) loses the plot (4,4)
20   Mesmerised for period near spring (10)
22   Hounds research facilities (4)
23   Caught actor Hathaway's film festival (6)
24   Close to a dozen per town show perseverance (8)

DOWN

1   Mannerism worst in midst of backstabbers (8)
2   Love 7-across? (4)
3   Corporation's last pay-cut to exhaust twit (10)
4   Tired go (4)
5   Asia copies corrupt stars (10)
6   Release *The French Journey* (3,3)
8   Vacuuming becoming obsolete? (9,4)
13   Skittish child genius snubbed one booking (10)
14   *Offspring* melody maintains climax (10)
16   Pacific island cocktail club feeding 11? (8)
18   Summit contracts top dogs (6)
21   Occupied coach at play's end (4)
22   Beat guitar flourish (4)

Puzzle 28 Friendly VIII

Beware of upcasing in 2-down, although not in 7-down, where I was sorely tempted to downcase . . .

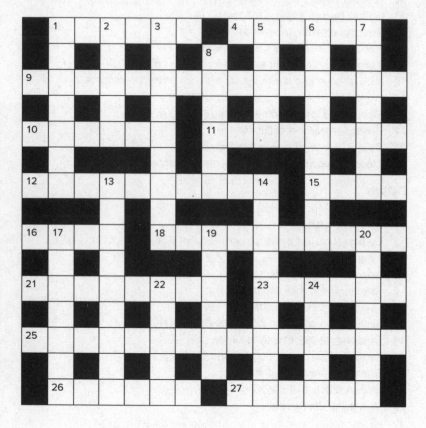

ACROSS

1   Merry company interrupts Joe's jig (6)
4   We became drug-free due to Skype tool? (6)
9   Filming drawing room? It's fair game (8,7)
10   Bank turned on inventor (6)
11   Food fanatic interchanged (8)
12   Fertilisers? They could be fit for a queen (10)
15   Belfast brigade question OPEC member (4)
16   Herb far from dill? (4)
18   She studies the divine tight/loose weave (10)
21   Heard to cut down box for crystalline mineral (8)
23   He waxed on high? (6)
25   Candid type likely to profit at 9-across (8,7)
26   Old man sees actress Fey in film (6)
27   My American 2-down in southern India (6)

DOWN

1   Toot almost suffices unknown male (4,3)
2   Ticked off Ford? (5)
3   Feral pets biting private silk producer (9)
5   Demand former law (5)
6   Two Manx dogs crashing (9)
7   Space station, plus NASA trailer, seen in *The Tempest*? (7)
8   Heard you look around African republic (6)
13   Dedicated to modify daft set as arrayed (9)
14   Greedily trade trimmed lace, discarded in dubious surrounds? (9)
17   One teacup-storm? Quiet! (3,2,2)
19   Blue records a feature of Canberra tavern? (6)
20   Significant other jam (7)
22   Heathen worship ending when I boycotted once more (5)
24   Many astonished ring (1,4)

Puzzle 29 Tricky I

Beware the curious twist on the alternation formula to open this new series. But otherwise a 'friendly' start to an evasive set coming your way.

ACROSS

1 Child-bearing yields Penny, oddly? (9)
6 Spike incorrect to change lead (5)
9 End of cacti pierced rambling peanut plant (7)
10 Book half-written by great biographer of Johnson (7)
11 Navigation tool consequently operated in reverse (5)
12 Angle to write? (4,1,4)
14 Covering most of 27-across (3)
15 Dismiss beauty as explosive (11)
17 Allergy trial to cancel cricket game (7,4)
19 Pagoda enshrines deity (3)
20 Dance till ruination of a romantic dinner (6-3)
22 Furtively examines grammatical roles (5)
24 Shackled, wearing mini, Ron stammered (2,5)
26 One footloose infant enters in the style of Persian hero (3,4)
27 Familiar parent, though backward (5)
28 Equals spy ring? (4,5)

DOWN

1 London diarist reported spies (5)
2 Obsolete SMS didn't start in court (7)
3 Troop Finn deployed for charity (3-6)
4 Original bloke broke head lantern (11)
5 Rearing son to be hooligan (3)
6 Kiss a Turkish official (5)
7 Original bloke is upright (7)
8 Midas' bloomer should he 12-across? (9)
13 Set up Whale Channel on air? (11)
14 Pain-loving chaos is rampant during 2000 (9)
16 Joining a tabaret, with a nude missing 14-down's pleasure? (9)
18 Wrought iron art displays rose (3,4)
19 Secret police cited in largest apology (7)
21 Eccentric concentric? (5)
23 Exchange about $1000 for bog (5)
25 Drain blood (3)

Puzzle 30 Tricky II

You'll notice a few more cross-references (as seen in 8-down), plus several spliced clues, such as 1-across. Welcome to the world of trickier puzzling.

ACROSS

1 See 28-across
5 Island apartment's ATM panels (3,4)
10 See 23-down
11 Plots for the late adversary corrupted by gangleader (10)
12 Snug to a pig dwelling (6)
13 He believes coach lit crackers (8)
14 Open to query a bed—strange piece of furniture (9)
16 Dog, parrots, hawks? (5)
19 Hurt with a safari knife (5)
21 Bulldozers reach into bankrupt city (9)
24 Flaunt high-fibre breakfast? (8)
25 Don't start please, OK (6)
27 Tom stopped charged routine (10)
28,1-across   Wine conventions near Papuan city (4,7)
29 Puts away short boundaries to gain cricketing prize (7)
30 Water source handy with odd tyre changes (7)

DOWN

2 Lionel overtly covering Marley classic (3,4)
3 Parramatta sounded out old Wallaby skipper (5)
4 SPECTRE swiped moneybag? (8)
6 Meets fair Eliot (6)
7 P-perfect sound of fog? (3-6)
8 Old man is at fault with 9-down, say (7)
9 Old lady madly curled belt-holder for painter (6,7)
14 Decline party food (3)
15 Jason's crew loves slang? Vice versa, we hear (9)
17 Spot unknown object (3)
18 Trash you'd recycle, losing nothing in island near 1-across (8)
20 Kinky pair on bed, pinkish . . . (7)
22 . . . yellow, bearing no end of outrage! (7)
23,10-across   Heroic Dickensian ringlet, we hear (6,4)
26 Light recorder? (5)

Puzzle 31 Tricky III

Zs, Js, Qs and Xs spice up several junctions in this grid. Use those rarities to your advantage.

ACROSS

8 Freezing quiet surrounds speaker and I (10)
9 Locks in Thai restaurant (4)
10 Turmoil disheartened paramour dreadfully . . . (6)
11 . . . in revised fling—adult rating libido (3,5)
12 Gosh! One quest radiated glamour (8)
13 Divers occasionally those who renege (6)
14 Sardonic one in Clancy (Overflow) (7)
16 Shot at bait (7)
19 Block my site: Puzzled (6)
21 Contrary skill by broadcaster ace, reaching puzzle's essence in Dixieland (4,4)
23 Outspoken eulogist not as high as Hawaiian volcano (5,3)
25 Pearl's house destroys terrible couches (6)
26 Slight object lost footing (4)
27 Uber-cool UK field can swing (10)

DOWN

1 Prop up handy tracks for purplish stone? (8)
2 Secretary gets short kid to cough up (3,3)
3 Frank almost 16? (4-6)
4 Goof to lament favourite getting up (7)
5 Big-screen finale dumped lead couple (4)
6 Native American female opens cola with end of knife (8)
7 Change pirate? (6)
13 Mathematician, on leaving snake forums? (10)
15 I get 2000 coin, very out-of-place in store (8)
17 Hurry up bizarre Zaire restaurant (8)
18 Overworks melodies (7)
20 Cheap platter carries silencer (6)
22 Jack regarding reddish quartz (6)
24 Raise 1554 cm? (4)

Puzzle 32 Tricky IV

You may need a 7-across to find all three puns clued here.

ACROSS

7   Organised defenders on borders offering this creature? (7,3)
9   See 21-down
10 Lattice current during Middle Ages? (6)
11 Prepare text in code, typo ruined on omission (8)
12 Jewel on axes (4)
13 Putting down infant with frog, jumping (10)
14 Clever dick sabotaged our helicopter (7,6)
17 Politician's primary place to be?! (10)
19 Registered meagre rain (4)
20 Blood-soaked hip instrument (8)
21 Negotiate healthy, saddled horse (6)
22,3-down   Soul music's Cooke to come again, before me too (4,4)
23 She barely rode into history! (4,6)

DOWN

1   Firmly fix gent doffing cap to outspoken jerk (8)
2   Left off-limits virus by outflow (6)
3   See 22-across
4   Study of lines in the sand? (10)
5   An obvious mammal feature is weird (not odd) on aardvark, say (8)
6   Stirring proposal (6)
8   Rubbed up tie and buckles lacking oomph? (13)
13 Generously diverted tuna by land (10)
15 Detailed flower sign on holy beads (8)
16 Soul mate? Right-o! (4-4)
18 Add more rounds to dire ordeal (6)
19 Every year, pusher quoted temple (6)
21,9-across   Cowboy's classic time for drawing? (4,4)

Puzzle 33   Tricky V

A long phrase, a dash of opera, philosophy, literature, dance, maths, business and greengrocery—all jammed into a 15 x 15 box.

ACROSS

1   Snake Sect perverted views (7)
5   Shattered glass at prison camps (7)
10,6-down   Hopeful glimpse, unless it's a 4-down (5,2,3,3,2,3,6)
11   *Revheads*, the opera? (6)
12   Underworld boss clipped main love poet (8)
13   Dance, then carols are broadcast (10)
15   Barge angles stern lower? (4)
16   Sounded appalling to sample vessel (4)
18   Rake leaf to grip ground (10)
20   'Bale' money for vintage Hollywood siren? (8)
22   Heavyweight gains edge over tea tycoon (6)
23   Slammin' Sam stereotyping basic software (9,6)
24   Vehement how decimals are calculated on bottom line (7)
25   Dutch humanist, at times, gets result 17-down (7)

DOWN

2   Leaves foreign cash to accommodate ATM requirement? (7)
3   Transient record linked to house's first Green, almost (9)
4   Coach's alternative coach? (5)
6   See 10-across
7   Tenor tours across Milan-Zaragoza (5)
8   Marx getting rough with company fraud? (7)
9   How countdowns proceed to be ruthless? (4,2,7)
14   Cockney lad loudly evaluates Asian flower (9)
15   Leo, say, dispatches pointers (9)
17   Bewildered tots climbing after final walls collapsed (2,1,4)
19   Going wild, author embracing ecstasy?! (7)
21   Inferior argument rejected servile ends (5)
22   Successful dieter or also-ran? (5)

Puzzle 34   Tricky VI

The quirky pattern alone should ring warning bells. This is one free-ranging puzzle. Enjoy the itinerary.

ACROSS

8   The way a Williams sister exchanged points (6)

9,2-down   French soldier to cry foul by Pole, having mountain-climbing worry (6,2,8)

10   Fairway feature to follow on (3-3)

11   Suits 14-across mare's gambol (8)

13   A gram wasted sweet wine, say, in aromatic mix (5,6)

14   Dictator's recognised novel (3)

15   Make out impasse in 11-across (7)

17   Helper reverted to drip method in Israel (3,4)

20   20-down short gown (3)

22   Mabo claim event? It lit a reform! (6,5)

24   Apes bishops (8)

25   Heading into Nauru brickworks (6)

26   US writer at funeral spree penned shock ending (8)

27   Pressure 21-down's neighbour, dispelling boisterous leader (4,2)

DOWN

1   Odd gear in designer jumper (8)

2   See 9-across

3   Function disrupts quiet historical building (6)

4   Engineering VIP cheery at barely resting (11)

5   Darn story related bogan hairstyle (4,4)

6,7-down   Way for British navy bloke to make beer, as heard in 17-across (6,6)

7   See 6-down

12   Dad possibly attended, he's stripping desk found here: (11)

16   Kits can't deploy the basics (3,5)

18   Old hands check mounted trap (8)

19   Asian guerrillas coveting skirmish (4,4)

20   Scam toilet paper procedure? (3-3)

21   Outspoken cove to exhaust capital (6)

23   Travelled to foreign sea after uni (6)

Puzzle 35   Tricky VII

I channelled my inner homie to create 15-down. And 'messive' apologies to any Kiwi solvers tackling 25-down.

ACROSS

1,11-across   Powerful athlete spinning girl with feet (6-6)
5   Preface return of prize article for nothing (8)
9   Student services wreaked havoc (15)
10   Twisting ponytail in fireplace (8)
11   See 1-across
12   *Maitre d'* welcoming turn to link seamlessly with hotel patron (5,5)
16   Lean inventory (4)
18   Harmony to sag in recital (4)
19   Hiker's device for one on trails? Pity (10)
22   See 3-down
24   Want hornet half-stabbing leg? (8)
26   Perhaps one did more Lit by crash course? (10,5)
27   Provide tucker outside the Tube? (8)
28   Blondes ignore interior layout (6)

DOWN

2   All examine veneer: highly surreal Boyd (9)
3,22-across   Announced restful street kid possibly producing
       rubbery gum? (5-6)
4   End of guilt trip results in flogging (7)
5   Adipose tissue, I guess, largely causes weariness (7)
6   Little flower fastener enclosing peeled bulb (7)
7   Turn cataracts into godsends? (9)
8   Girl intermittently skipped troop-ship to attend marine base (5)
13   Snarled at clock, wearing quiet garment for penitent (9)
14   Guru in casino finishes card game (3)
15   'Yo! Have a drink.' (3)
17   Cake pan or vanity case? (6,3)
19   Old Roman wheels spy into bed (7)
20   Less clear how Scrooge held it aloft (7)
21   Embellished hearing began after attorney's opener (7)
23   Rising fame nearly interrupted medical procedure (5)
25   Hikes with NZ fools by sound (5)

Puzzle 36   Tricky VIII

At first glance, this puzzle may seem closer to a Friendly grading. Until you try solving it. Fact is, I'm getting you 23-across for the Gnarly finale!

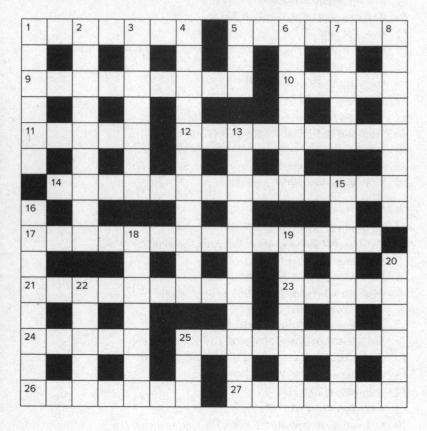

ACROSS

1 Last month, our foremost spirit dignified behaviour (7)
5 Indonesian island almost repelled river missile (7)
9 Grating quality vexed city nerds (9)
10 Brave partner belittled team win (5)
11 Stripped ego should expose demon (5)
12 Extolled outstanding court expert (9)
14 New Yorkers hugely drug-injected for delicate operation (7,7)
17 The wages of sin? (3-6,5)
21 Beg 'Peter' of fiction, perhaps (9)
23 Prepared fresh rye sandwiches and sides (5)
24 I get loud sticker from Arctic shelter? (5)
25 Trace call—it's in disarray (9)
26 Felt excitement when model socialised topless? (7)
27 Botch email in steamy gym? (7)

DOWN

1 Style pundit prescribed intake (6)
2 Physical reef structure surrounds small hole (9)
3 Sport swimmer dropping in to see Santa's helper (7)
4 Guillotine followed, absorbing terrible pain when used (11)
5 Glee just on your faces? (3)
6 Six (or it's sixes and sevens) for guest (7)
7 Yahoos lowered water-flower's pith (5)
8 Renegade nods away of late (8)
13 Somehow outer Brisbane seems anti-truancy (11)
15 Odd reminder prepared way for literary hoax of 1944 (3,6)
16 Locate code objective (8)
18 Where you may find butter running hot? (2,1,4)
19 Makes bubbly seawater, curiously lacking tungsten (7)
20 Pirate's agreement to audit two in old Rome? (3-3)
22 Gown's hem stitched—only synthetic? (5)
25 Showing up my blue (3)

Puzzle 37   Gnarly I

If you find the jump to Gnarly too great, then peek at one solution, and work backwards. But only after your brain's been truly stretched. (Please note: 28-across rates among the bluest clues you've met. And toughest.)

ACROSS

1 Fruit close to sandwiches, a vessel (5,4)
6 Midget firework (5)
9 Battles to retain war's prime witnesses (5)
10 Stud had wanton wife start to pause (3,3,3)
11 It's cutting geek and fiend into shreds (5-4)
12 Grim reference linked back to nuclear physicist (5)
13 Staff not going hungry with a thick porridge? (7)
15 Ridiculed smeared edges holding short latte (7)
17 Bill pockets $11 roughly for Uber rival (7)
19 British actor delivers foul talk to Spooner (4,3)
20 Drug hidden in shoe? (5)
22 Collectively solve after first squall (9)
25 Curse Angola unrest involving six sides (9)
26 Fear mid-April comes in late (5)
27 Big O transposed Greek finale (5)
28 Groovy skirts, minus rough stuff from quickie? (4,5)

DOWN

1 Brief month (and a weekend) with 1950s sex-bomb (5)
2 Renovated places fix movie art (7,2)
3 Offspring debate (5)
4 Spiky customer sees comical dame clutching cross in Athens (7)
5 Misled emperor's starting off in baby clothing (7)
6 Calm if dragons clawed (9)
7 Drug dealers shelled theatre employee (5)
8 Kid's doggie holds in dog lead in building protrusion (3,6)
13 Badgers touchier after park gets shrew-tamer (9)
14 Hurryin' up cat endlessly below Honduras (9)
16 Sheep, perhaps, frustrate one missing cows, perhaps (9)
18 Second-class report of sarcasm of *Don Juan* poet (7)
19 American can bound one with superb sport (3,4)
21 Fairy 9 or 11 broke baker's dish (5)
23 Mongrel mantra corrupted city (5)
24 Dwarf to introduce himself to wine? (5)

Puzzle 38 Gnarly II

One answer owns 38 letters, making it a very handy answer to get.

ACROSS

1   Dutch cheese I omitted to bind 'stew (7)
5   Old communicator firm enlisted Pitt and me (1.1.,5)
10   Egoistic bunch subject classes to in-fighting (3,2,10)
11   See 22-across
12   Dead Centre in torments with the high temperature (5,4)
14   Liquid regrettably inadequate—it keeps stocking up (6,4)
15   Online lair promised land? (4)
16,4-down   Spooner's 'C on 9' a luminous message (4,4)
18   Needles crochet tan garment (6,4)
20   Dizzy? Breather saw dizziness initially go (9)
22,11-across   Offer stock to common-sounding aircraft (5,5)
24,9-down,6-down   Could be worse, compared to campfire accident?
       (6,4,1,4,2,3,3,4,1,5,5)
25   Mark Twain, maybe, put lamb heart in pasta (3-4)
26   Thousands of refugees originally flee shackles (7)

DOWN

2   Crude oil heap drowning in dramatic circumstances? (7)
3   Hollywood dynasty gain weight due to cake? (9)
4   See 16-across
6   See 24-across
7   A bug often neglected in East London (5)
8   Mission ignored odds and departed strand (7)
9   See 24-across
13   Treated the rust, adding strange sodium pentothal (5,5)
15   Gums signal up, sending semaphore essentially into anarchic Italy (9)
17   Curse Livy medley with pronounced ease (4,3)
19   Regrettably able to audit North American (7)
21   Divulge heading for language school near Windsor (3,2)
23   Girl planned occupation (4)

Puzzle 39   Gnarly III

Watch out for two intricate deletion recipes, both of the Down persuasion. And that's the only hint you're getting.

ACROSS

1 Treasonous crime exploited greed, here in French parts (8)
5 Just a diagram demonstrating sporting venues (6)
10 Elder bear mauling waist of Pontiff (5)
11 1-across in 19-across, OK, pal? (9)
12 Husky goods Mike shifted (6,3)
13 Loves penning name of NZ peninsula (5)
14 Desert omen I mentioned (5)
16 Diner's alternative to crow? (6,3)
18 Freak or TV model – he can't be named (9)
19 Snores first and last after a 'blanking' long musical—. . . (5)
21 . . .—hence my mixers (5)
23 Try one show, *Carousel* (9)
26 Expanded on a Dobell redraft (9)
27 Avoid state taxes up-front (5)
28 Communiques regressively ooze over article (6)
29 Zone evacuated often, linked to really extreme fanaticism (8)

DOWN

1 Murderous Jack's beauties? (7)
2 Cossack steps set off stuff, we hear (5)
3 Harlequin's love to skip canoe stern under short pier (9)
4 Doesn't start cold cut (5)
6 Capital to knowingly shell Cambodian hub (5)
7 Smooth over sufficient evidence (1.1.1.,6)
8 A starfish points to rockpool resident! (7)
9 Oil a saw below mountain (8)
15 Stunning lead inlet of Egypt! (4,5)
16 Fool pirate nursing bad wind (8)
17 Lite shout doesn't cost much (5,4)
18 Even Princess quit, that's plain (7)
20 Pretty narrowly lost crucial final (7)
22 Damage hole blocking upward rims (5)
24 Low-budget film to show cat missing? (5)
25 Tree near top of grove suffering hail (5)

Puzzle 40 Gnarly IV

That *regular brain* (see 10-across) will get a proper workout with this cocktail of innovation and manipulation. The hardest clue you've met so far could be 15-across.

ACROSS

1 Sorry a mallet-wielding guy evacuated? (7)
5 Unspeakable Scottish king (7)
10 Period in regular brain unravelling communications obstacle (8,7)
11 Banjo-plucking rap notes? (8)
12 Newly arrange holiday destination (6)
13 Are chauvinists endless? (5)
15 Was possibly overanxious? (4,5)
17 Polish worker down at heel? (9)
19 Flips photos (5)
22 Cockney's 18-down warmer in winter? (6)
23 Chronically hassled, I promote salad (4-4)
25 How Gandhi turned to Mama instantaneously? (2,3,4,2,1,3)
26 A nozzle leads into limited refined gas (7)
27 Tolerate bread basket (7)

DOWN

2 Troop of alpha rebels meet next regulars (7)
3 Theatre box conceals one TV award (5)
4 Changed sides in smooth green? (6)
6 Willingness in the style of urbanised Romeo? (8)
7 Mug supports capital composer (9)
8 Dance, sculpture etc to suit tango foremost (3,4)
9 Cherry almost in bloom for second cosmic bite? (13)
14 Hazy tapes show illegal factory (9)
16 Irish playwright brasher, I'd announce in part (8)
18 Pouch strapped to chest of drawers? (7)
20 Jeep tail hits Cairo's pedestrian (7)
21 Introduce significance (6)
24 Song lines ultimately in hand (5)

Puzzle 41 Gnarly V

Pedants may quibble with the US spelling of 8-down, despite the same version dominating menus and shop signs. (That's why the clue's surface sense feels extra fitting.)

ACROSS

1 Defaced shelters in shady spots (7)
5 Jacked-up hedonist ripping nylon top off (7)
9 Holy Father quit grand finale (3)
10 Press pursued audio scam—a torch job? (7,4)
11 Arranges queues (5,2)
12 Pot belly? (4,3)
14 Aware of blue-bereted Teletubby? (2,2)
15 Contest charge implicating reputation we own (10)
18 See 13-down
21 Celebrity constituent of 4-down (4)
23 Country behind detaining the Spanish soldier (7)
24 Less vivid instant in Sicily (7)
25 Buffalo, salmon, tiger, lizard (4,7)
27 Pick up Native American? (3)
28 He painted young girls, barely wearing a shirt (7)
29 Farms opened outlets (7)

DOWN

1 Hallucinogen tangled us in knots (5,4)
2 Scouts' trailblazer to study force, contracted to implant blast (5-6)
3 Campuses accept point after point, none too savvy (6)
4 Sign 20 − 1 + 3.142 + 0 (7)
5 Jumpers face this, drugged at pub (4,3)
6 Filmed 9th ace, remarkably? (2,3,3)
7 21-across uncapped pitch (3)
8 Blow stack over sweet nothing? (5)
13,18-across   Perfunctorily examines proposals? (4,7,3,7)
16 Baker's treats in pot maverick strove to seal (9)
17 Pop pianist bewitching to Maoris (4,4)
19 Big blokes penetrated semi-wild (7)
20 Regrets panning some flip file-sharing scheme of the noughties (7)
22 Old-money resort, no-frills once lands are cleared? (6)
23 Heck, jolly swagman's campsite! (2,3)
26 Parcel collection (3)

Puzzle 42   Gnarly VI

How are these gnarly puzzles treating you? Still 27-across through the clues, or are you due to 9-down?

ACROSS

1 Pervert to express pleasure, reclining in bed (7)
5 Stand in partial vault of Talmud school (7)
10 Butcher offering return of party snacks (6,4)
11 Squarish lad steals kiss (4)
12 Horse tricks lose rider, flanks trapped (6)
13 Tires of khaki? (8)
14 Ned custom-made files (9)
16,18-across   Ink producer grants right to capitulate for one pound (5,5)
18 See 16-across
20 One played blues on radio for recruits (9)
23 Orange truck transports the French spies (8)
24 Shred organ during setback (4,2)
26 War god methodically dispensed fairness (4)
27 Wild pastry-stealing initially ignored (10)
28 July's session samples Joyce's work (7)
29 Risk gobbling chocolate bar that's neither here nor there (7)

DOWN

2 Wheel firm admits iron deficiency in river (7)
3 Okay bloke? (5)
4,15-down   C O S M O S
            C O S M O S (8,9)
6 Modernise energetic tryst (6)
7 Friendship embraces Ukraine leader? It can be read two ways (9)
8 Devoid of church, existence turned square (7)
9 Dope rites half-adjusted to lose control (2,3,3,5)
15 See 4-down
17 Quick-tempered soul leans over sack (8)
19 Dispute leadlight piece (7)
21 Regarding horse skipping last bullock in even time (7)
22 Dubious 26-across gets 200 in short supply (6)
25 Wonky request we upheld (5)

Puzzle 43   Gnarly VII

Four extended entries in this puzzle, plus two lengthy spliced clues. When ahas arrive, the grid could well fill fast.

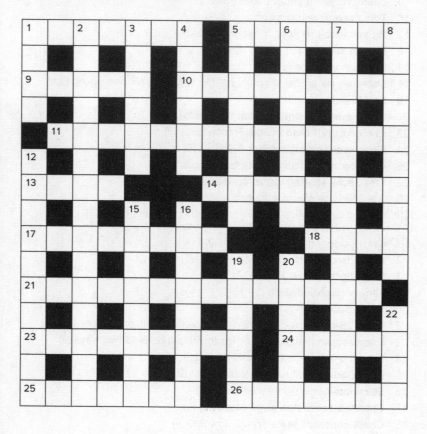

ACROSS

1 Sikh wraps dry on reflection, needing occasional garnish (7)
5 Cheat German woman in half-hearted act (7)
9 Lizard, wagtail, parrot by the sounds (5)
10 Turn to cover address and vanish (9)
11 Tabloid excess is almost insane mischief (14)
13 Find over-neglected platter (4)
14,22-down Versatile tuber blew the mood apart (2.,6,4)
17 Man *is* an island, thanks to this! (5,3)
18 Hellish Belleville quartet (4)
21 Listen carefully—grog went to mend misery (4,3,2,5)
23 Cop impounds drug in these? (5,4)
24 Cheer the football drama at the finals (5)
25 Compiler hacked a test fact-file (4,3)
26 Clot where angels proverbially dance (7)

DOWN

1,6-down Travel part of West Africa for mob at fault (2,2,4,1,2,1)
2 Genius flogged corniest tickets (6,9)
3 A trick to oxygenate fire (6)
4 Some hussies take 20 winks? (6)
5 Yard once prepared for clergy (8)
6 See 1-down
7 Twice 25-across with vegan—is curiously left with few choices (2,1,12)
8 Armed criminal twisted so-called theme park (10)
12 Journo spin opening up Dickensian (5,5)
15 John Clarke spoof, say, wounding English banker (3,5)
16 Electorate hit on safety measure (4-4)
19 Cat lifted iron first to spill beans (4,2)
20 Comic cousin of 14-across 22-down? (2.,4)
22 See 14-across

Puzzle 44 Gnarly VIII

More than a few anagrams here, so maybe I didn't save the gnarliest till last?
Only one way for you to find out . . .

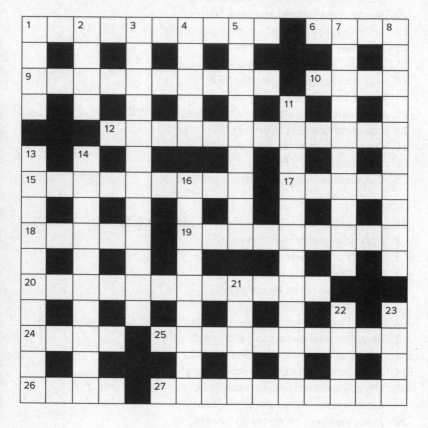

ACROSS

1 ABC's creepy new computer network (10)
6 Excited nuclear pedagogues (4)
9 Complex on a 'phut' IBM instrument (5,5)
10 Bordering on desperate, joining second rally (4)
12 In kitchen, note holder of farm egg I'd scramble—clear? (6-6)
15 Grab bung to obstruct stupid lawn problem (4,5)
17 Otologist tedium? (5)
18 A tailed toy losing tail to a dog (5)
19 Blind sample discrimination at big match (5,4)
20 Perhaps KGB cops get erectile dysfunction (6,6)
24 Vegetable box gets Oliver's head spinning (4)
25 Give Penny debt (10)
26 Don't touch hat kid tossed (4)
27 Plum fortune is squandered, given time (5,5)

DOWN

1 How to make time, Tim, dear? (4)
2 Start off regarding match (4)
3 Poet from interior makes appeal to host arty-sounding parties (6,6)
4 Enquired into Lions group invoice? (5)
5 Accord to swindle head count at hearing (9)
7 British commando gets reminder before welcome clasps (5,5)
8 Pen for another—turns hackneyed in recital (5-5)
11 Help end off gutter with main wiper (12)
13 1900 dissonant shelled deplorably large residences (10)
14 Horse remedy I swallowed twice for chemist? (5,5)
16 It can help plane loop it, perhaps, following a sporadic gust (9)
21 Study nonsense poet, Nash (not Wood)? (5)
22 Place where officer evicted tenant (4)
23 Centre of attention, though not a positive in Moscow (4)

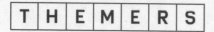

Puzzle 45 Themer I

These last six puzzles come with a theme, or carry instructions that influence the clues in some way. Let's begin with a mild 'themer' owning a subset of interconnecting answers.

ACROSS

1 Boy's finishing for love in current style, usually (9)
6 Spotted one laughing aboard dinghy, enamoured (5)
9 *Grease*—the painting? (3)
10 Flavour source available, processed with fennel core (7,4)
11 After 51, count bungled print design (7)
12 Photographic pioneer guy beside the point (7)
14 Sack Labour fizgig (8)
16 It has ears—half ears—and a bit of eye (6)
18 Love commercial muck (6)
19 Alcoholic radical led a nasty, fiendish mister (8)
21 Girl is confusing aces with jack (7)
22 Unravel at Xmas time when drunk, we hear (7)
25 Organic supply shop came top for mulching (7,4)
27 Briefly pursue old invader (3)
28 Partial stratagem most rejected in battle (5)
29 Van Gogh had this biscuit (6,3)

DOWN

1 Fish a pest on line? (5)
2 13-down star finally visited city's 7-down, 24-down, 26-down and . . . (11)
3 . . . municipal figures known to Caesar (5)
4 Pneumonoultramicroscopicsilicovolcanoconiosis is chronic! (4-4)
5 Cried out deeply (6)
6 Jewel in *The Crown* a plot marker? (9)
7 Examine tuber bud (3)
8 A nun discontented with beer in Sydney's inner west (9)
13 May, say, hold one call from 1-across, regarding old comic troupe (5,6)
14 Wave lifts pancakes (9)
15 Line-up, maybe, is more disturbing (9)
17 Sponge on club (8)
20 Explorer announced passion to travel north (6)
23 Wood fuzz mentioned (5)
24 Edict withstanding revolution (5)
26 She has a change of heart in America (3)

Puzzle 46 Themer II

Here's our first encounter with a standfirst—the crossword-term for any instructions sitting above the puzzle's clues. As you'll read, all Across answers are related, and thus their clues avoid any definition. (Hence wiser solvers will attack the Down clues first.)

(NB: Answers to all Across clues share a theme, and go otherwise undefined. Down clues are normal.)

ACROSS

8 Alpha twice interrupts Mr Average? (8)
9 Is dramatic 19-down retrograde? (6)
10 Backed one household cleaner (4)
11 Pole-axe rebel leader during another struggle (5,5)
12 Drug and Alcohol Unit (6)
14 Smooth 24-down capering within (8)
15 Arteries stemmed injury (7)
17 An animated explorer on podcast? (7)
20 Gets this copy bias universally trimmed (8)
22 Zipper heard? (6)
23 Report lashed out (10)
24 Aqualung discovered (4)
25 Criminal core grasps one rule (6)
26 Model helper holds boxer back (8)

DOWN

1 Literary recluse needing walls in beleaguered 9-across (8)
2 A pointless 25-across leads to . . . (4)
3 . . . themed entry coin (6)
4 Tree announcing another themed entry (7)
5 Aristocratic Spooner to purchase trumpet (4-4)
6 Sweet cereal of poor lost rogue? (5,5)
7 RGN in sound or sea? (6)
13 Hood's hood? (10)
16 Misshape blurry focus (8)
18 Brainstorms plus storm front (4,4)
19 A gag implicit in this compiler's grandeur (7)
21 It dangles a graduate in costume, cryptically (3-3)
22 Are the cooks to prepare leftovers? (6)
24 Pass trainer's first horse (4)

Puzzle 47   Themer III

If you're unfamiliar with 19-across, this puzzle may beat you. Then again, every related clue gives you the raw material you need for success . . .

ACROSS

1 A harvest (and what may store it) seen from behind Greek temple (9)
6 Dated writer virtually encaged a bird (5)
9 A daughter to 5-down emerged (5)
10 Two-thirds of season fulfilling old Greek writer of 19-across (3,6)
11 13-down's eldest oddly ❤ couple? (6)
12 She constantly disputes ice-breaker breaking off metal now and then (8)
14 5-down's middle child (cruel sot) left 19-across destitute (3)
16 Strew ill-skewered herbicides (11)
19 Novel influence deters rupture internally (11)
20 Yoghurt brand to go downhill (3)
21 Fans err terribly, wearing Proteas cap showing coarse plant (4,4)
23 11-across's sister lives in denial, eating the wrong way (6)
26 Supports tether/ . . . (9)
27 . . . or paddock fences removed by 13-down's wife (5)
28 Linger, exchanging ring for a partner of 5-down (5)
29 Mini-vehicle has a cruel prang involving three bees in the air? (6,3)

DOWN

1 Papa (the ticklish lodger) lacking interest (9)
2 Sit for torso, bust (5)
3 Took an early look, and quietly criticised . . . (9)
4 . . . topless Fonda film, with strings attached? (4)
5 Power grass-cutters without 19-across patriarch (3,7)
6 Prompt 13-down's son (5)
7 Lawyers at contests ousting upstart (9)
8 Recluse more akin to 13-down's first son? (5)
13 19-across patriarch arranged trees among shops, over brick veneer (6,4)
15 Flaky coal drips, carrying excess fluid? (9)
17 Oil-well model twice blasted slight European hooter (6,3)
18 He whines to vendor keeping French wine skyrocketing? (9)
21 6-down's sister getting old boy dressed (5)
22 Suspicious of 19-across survivor? (5)
24 Hearts of resilient Saracens touching on hip? (5)
25 22-down son to 5-down? (4)

Puzzle 48   Themer IV

Not just a standfirst, this puzzle also owns several rule-pushing clues (such as 8-across and 15-across), making this teaser as tortuous (and torturous) as they come.

(NB: Answers to all the Across clues share a theme, and go otherwise undefined. Down clues are normal.)

ACROSS

 8 Large axe? (8)
 9 Model wearing bright . . . (6)
10 . . . retro belt (4)
11 Regular guys (men) had set pieces (10)
12 Debate losing steam from the outset (6)
14 Disorderly 2-down 24-down (8)
15 Candy stick? (7)
17 Crookedly handling barbed-wire? (7)
20 Strip booty for Spooner (8)
22 Money-clip in Job Centre (6)
23 Linen wasn't crumpled (4,6)
24 Gutless 17-across move (4)
25 A speed beyond 1000 (6)
26 Square legs (8)

DOWN

 1 Most stick up for city leaders fleeing (8)
 2 23-across force detailed payola (4)
 3 Ways to finish snags? (6)
 4 Lee's aim deviated 1829 metres (3-4)
 5 Adventure excites on vacation, getting a dwelling within castle walls (8)
 6 Feature of Cagney's angels and ribald fire-front experts (5,5)
 7 Tax accounts lack an over-the-top application (6)
13 Harry, Alice, Donna, Scot (10)
16 Cleaned up a perfect score, destitute? (8)
18 Figures smooch, soon head over heels! (8)
19 Call centre abandoned, having reported duplication (7)
21 A crude vessel carrying a Palestinian statesman, once (6)
22 Returned aboard airman's second plane (6)
24 Cut drug run (4)

Puzzle 49 Themer V

Some clues are starred this time, while the grid has its own instructions. No wonder this crossword occupies the book's pointy end. Look both ways!

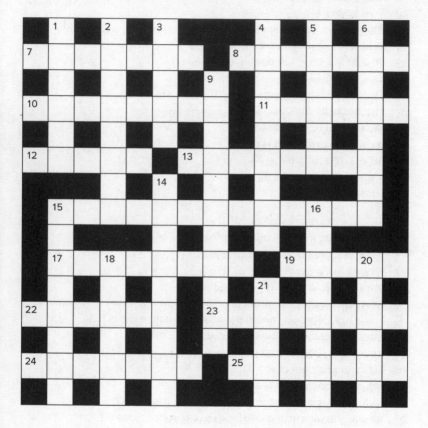

(NB: You must solve 15-across before entering related answers to the starred clues, each lacking a definition element.)

ACROSS

*7 Expecting a replacement for tenderfoot (7)

*8 Crank letters (7)

10 Lure to give line distortion (8)

11 Copper plus iodine contributing to weird radioactive element (6)

12 Devotee's heart forbidding bouquet (5)

*13 Some music I do, I represent revolution (8)

15 Avenge her talents, but fail (4,3,6)

17 Obedient blokes in detox group depressed to miss turn (8)

*19 Sailor initially jettisoned bark's contents (5)

*22 Hit the smorgasbord? (6)

23 Mutant spawning bird feature (8)

*24 Mystical Orient's interior (7)

*25 Spanish mackerel catcher? (7)

DOWN

*1 Guessing four (or six) off (6)

*2 Minor law, say (8)

3 Ends of purer merino improving class jumpers? (5)

4 Chisels lop back a Hill End gem (5,4)

5 Unlimited sum steadier for Shylock (6)

6 Wins shirt worn to cover ref (8)

*9 The Spanish doctor I'm joining in Wild West (6-5)

14 Way-out side stole paddle-wheeler (9)

15 Plane figures pin up 25-across material after facelifts (8)

*16 Suspect falls? Boo! (8)

*18 One orally spluttered upon?! (6)

20 Cottoned on fast, grasping either Karl Marx essence (6)

21 Virtuous harpist, in fury, swapped hands (5)

Puzzle 50   Themer VI

What theme would you deem a dream conclusion for *Rewording the Brain*?

(To reword your brain, the letters occupying the shaded squares will be over-looked by their respective clues' wordplay. Every other clue is normal.)

ACROSS

1 Fresh against Christmas season wrapping (5)
4 Hotspots? They order locks (9)
9 We contribute to online workshop (7)
10 Rank desserts, reviewed with hesitation (7)
11 Like piranha lessening shock on one exposed bank (9)
12 It's essential to test opinion! (5)
13 Boring years, twice losing energy in prison (6)
15 Finally you had to loosen locks (7)
17 He made a scale more loaded, carrying ton (7)
19 Revealing bigfoot (6)
22 Contemporarily oppose poetry? (5)
23 Darned pro in spin?! (3,6)
25 Outflow edging sort of trout? (7)
26 12-across mentioned Audrey Hepburn's title role (7)
27 Incessant greediness sadly raging (6,3)
28 Oz painter nearly owns odds to make comeback (5)

DOWN

1 1-across piece for Seinfeld character (6)
2 Electrifying box from below (7)
3 Perversely love to try language (5)
4 Larger university shredded *Herald*? (9)
5 Playwright unmasked writers on Central Avenue (5)
6 Barer grub (fritters) here?! (6,3)
7 Girl picked up a summery glow at quiet end of Cronulla (7)
8 Siberian dogs wagged some days (8)
14 Flaming seabird crossing Black Island to waste vessels (6,3)
15 Made for the city, unlike 1-across (9)
16 OT book favouring rock and roll, for example (8)
18 Unloaded cartridge firearm (7)
20 Tricked up Latin for wedding . . . (7)
21 . . . or European-sounding decree (6)
23 Make peace with Scottish distiller? (5)
24 Former Israeli PM offers nothing cryptic! (5)

S O L U T I O N S

| F | O | R | M | U | L | A | | K | E | Y | |

*	anagram
+	charade
[ ]	container
<	reversal
alt	alternation
code	code
dd	double definition
ex/AMPLE	deletion
hid	hidden
man	manipulation
pun	aka cryptic definition
'quay'	homophone
reb	rebus
spoon	spoonerism

Puzzle 1 solution

D	A	N	E		T	H	U	S

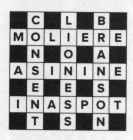

ACROSS
1 DANE* (not DEAN!)
3 THUS*
7 PIROUETTE*
8 STEAMIRON*
9 THIRSTIER*
10 DINE*
11 USED*

DOWN
1 DEPOSITED*
2 NORWEGIAN*
4 HITORMISS*
5 SEEINGRED*
6 SURMISE*

Puzzle 2 solution

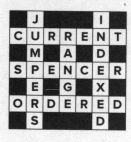

ACROSS
4 MOLIERE [hid]
5 ASININE [hid]
6 IN A SPOT [hid]

DOWN
1 CONSENT [hid]
2 LIONESS [hid]
3 BRANSON [hid]

Puzzle 3 solution

ACROSS
3 CURRENT [dd]
5 SPENCER [dd]
6 ORDERED [dd]

DOWN
1 JUMPERS [dd]
2 INDEXED [dd]
4 RANGE [dd]

Puzzle 4 solution

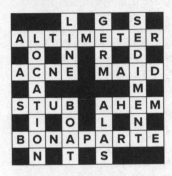

P	A	C	E			E	M	M	A
A		A		M		E			D
R	E	T	R	E	A	T	E	D	
C		A		L		R			R
H	O	M	E	A	L	O	N	E	
M		A		N		N			S
E	G	R	E	G	I	O	U	S	
N		A		E		M			E
T	A	N	K			H	E	R	D

ACROSS
1 P+ACE
3 E+M+MA
7 RE+TREAT+ED
8 HO+MEAL+ONE
9 E+GREG+IOUS
10 TAN+K
11 HER+D

DOWN
1 P+ARCH+MEN+T
2 CAT+A+MAR+A+N
4 MET+RON+O+ME
5 A+D+DRESSED
6 ME+LANGE

Puzzle 5 solution

		L		G		S	
A	L	T	I	M	E	T	E	R
	O		N		R		D
A	C	N	E		M	A	I	D
	A						M
S	T	U	B		A	H	E	M
	I		O		L		N
B	O	N	A	P	A	R	T	E
	N		T		S	

ACROSS
4 AL[TIME]TER
6 AC[N]E
7 MA[I]D
8 S[T]UB
10 A[HE]M
11 BON[APART]E

DOWN
1 LI[N]E
2 GE[R]M
3 SE[DIME]NT
5 LO[CA]TION
9 B[O]AT
10 A[LA]S

Puzzle 6 solution

	M		L		S	
P	A	L	E	T	T	E
	T		D		O	
H	A	N	G	E	R	S
	D		E		I	
B	O	A	R	D	E	R
	R		S		S	

ACROSS
4 'PALETTE'
5 'HANGERS'
6 'BOARDER'

DOWN
1 'MATA'+'DOR'
  ['matter+door']
2 'LEDGERS'
3 'STORIES'

Puzzle 7 solution

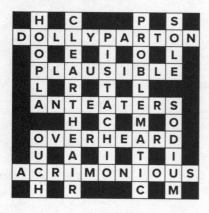

ACROSS

1 SPOTS [dd]
4 STOPS*
8 BEAN+COUNTER [dd]
9 FILL+ET
10 SPIN<
11 STUD/y
12 ICECAP [hid]
13 GRASSHOPPER [dd]
15 SCARE*
16 'CRATE'

DOWN

2 PREHISTORIC*
3 TANG+LED
5 TEN [alt]
6 PREDIC[AMEN]T
7 'FORT'+'NIGHT'
10 SLEEPER [dd]
14 SIR [code]

Puzzle 8 solution

ACROSS

5 DOLLY+PART+ON
7 PLAUSIBLE*
8 d/ANTE+c/ATERS
10 OVER+'HEARD'
11 ACRIMONIOUS*

DOWN

1 HOOP-LA [dd]
2 CLEARTHEAIR*
3 PROBLEMATIC*
4 'SOLE'
6 PISTACHIO*
9 S+ODIUM
10 c/OUCH

Puzzle 9 solution

P	A	I	R		T		A	S	I	A
E		N		D	A	B		P		P
C	A	T	E	R	P	I	L	L	A	R
K		R		A		L		I		O
S	P	A	S	M		L	A	T	I	N
		V		A	H	A		S		
T	W	E	E	T		B	R	E	A	D
I		N		I		O		C		R
G	R	O	S	S	I	N	C	O	M	E
E		U		T	A	G		N		A
R	O	S	E		N		A	D	A	M

ACROSS
1 'PAIR'
4 AS+IA
7 DAB<
9 CATER+PILLAR
10 S[PAS]M [alt]
11 LATIN [hid]
12 AHA<
13 T+WEE+T
14 'BREAD'
16 GROSS INCOME [rebus]
18 TAG [dd]
19 p/ROSE
20 A+DAM<

DOWN
1 'PECKS'
2 INTRAVENOUS [hid]
3 TAP [dd]
5 SPLIT+SECOND
6 A[PRO]N
7 DRAM+AT+IST
8 BILL+A+BONG
13 TIGER [code]
15 D[RE]AM
17 I+AN

Puzzle 10 solution

T	A	K	E	T	H	E	C	A	K	E
A		I		I	X		N		N	N
D	E	N	I	M		C	A	D	E	T
		D		E	E		E			R
B	R	E	A	S	T	P	L	A	T	E
R		S		S	T		V			E
A	N	T	I	Q	U	I	T	I	E	S
C			U		O		G			
K	A	P	P	A		N	I	N	T	H
E		I		R		A		O		A
N	E	T	H	E	R	L	A	N	D	S

ACROSS
1 TAKE THE CAKE [pun]
7 DENIM<
8 CAD+ET
9 BREASTP*+LATE
11 ANTIQUITIES*
12 'KAPPA'
14 NINTH [hid]
16 NET+HERLANDS*

DOWN
1 TA+D
2 KIN+DEST/ined
3 TIMES SQUARE [reb]
4 EXCEPTIONAL*
5 h/AND
6 g/ENT+f/REEs
9 BRACKEN*
10 AVI*+GNON<
13 PIT [dd]
15 HAS [dd]

Puzzle 11 solution

R	I	F	L	E		P	I	C	A	S
A		E		M		A		H		T
C	O	N	T	E	M	P	L	A	T	E
E		C		R		E		N		A
D	U	E		A	C	R	O	N	Y	M
		S		L		W		E		
D	W	I	N	D	L	E		L	A	P
O		T		C		I		S		E
S	I	T	T	I	N	G	D	U	C	K
E		E		T		H		R		E
S	T	R	A	Y		T	O	F	F	S

ACROSS

1 RIFLE*
4 PICAS/so
7 CON+TEMPL[AT]E
8 DUE [dd]
9 A+CRONY+M
10 DWINDLE [hid]
11 LAP [dd]
13 SITTING+DUCK
14 ST[R]AY
15 TOFFS [hid]

DOWN

1 t/RACED
2 FENCE SITTER [spoon]
3 EMERALDCITY*
4 P+APER+'WEIGHT'
5 CHANNEL-SURF [pun]
6 STEAM [code]
10 DO[S]ES
12 PEKES*

Puzzle 12 solution

U	S	A	G	E		S	W	I	F	T
	T		A		S		A		I	
P	E	T	S	E	M	A	T	A	R	Y
	P		P		A		C		E	
G	H	O	S	T	S		H	O	S	T
	E			S	H			T		
S	N	A	G		H	I	T	M	A	N
	K		R		I		I		R	
D	I	R	E	S	T	R	A	I	T	S
	N		E		S		R		E	
A	G	E	N	T		C	A	R	R	Y

ACROSS

1 U+SAGE [alt]
4 SWIFT [dd]
8 PETS<+EMATARY*
9 G[HOST]S
10 HOST [dd]
11 SNAG [man]
13 w/HITMAN
15 DIRESTRAITS*
16 AGE+NT
17 'CARRY'

DOWN

2 STEP+HEN+KING
3 G+ASPS
5 WATCH [pun]
6 FIRESTARTER*
7 SMASH HITS [smashing HITS makes THIS]
12 G[RE]EN
14 TIARA [hid]

Puzzle 13 solution

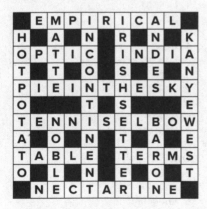

P	O	K	E	R		B	I	K	E	R
L		L		E		A		I		O
A	G	E	N	T	O	R	A	N	G	E
S		P		I		D		D		
M	U	T	I	N	Y		C	H	I	P
A		O		A		S		E		A
S	U	M	O		A	U	P	A	I	R
		A		H		P		R		S
F	U	N	D	A	M	E	N	T	A	L
O		I		K		R		E		E
G	H	A	N	A		B	I	D	D	Y

ACROSS

1 POKER [dd]
4 BI/g+KER/b
7 A+GENT+O+RANGE
8 MU/st+TINY
9 CHIP [dd]
12 SUM+O
13 AU+PAIR [pun]
15 FUND+A+MENTAL
16 'GHANA'
17 BIDDY* [minus O]

DOWN

1 PLA+SMAS<
2 KLEPTOMANIA [pun]
3 RETINA [hid]
4 BARD<
5 KINDHEARTED*
6 'ROE'
10 PARSLEY*
11 SU[PER]B
14 HAKA [code]
15 F+OG<

Puzzle 14 solution

	E	M	P	I	R	I	C	A	L	
H		A		N		R		N		K
O	P	T	I	C		I	N	D	I	A
T		T		O		S		E		N
P	I	E	I	N	T	H	E	S	K	Y
O				T		S		S		E
T	E	N	N	I	S	E	L	B	O	W
A		O		N		T		A		E
T	A	B	L	E		T	E	R	M	S
O		L		N		E		O		T
	N	E	C	T	A	R	I	N	E	

ACROSS

1 EMPIRICAL*
8 OPTIC*
9 INDIA [hid &lit]
10 PIE IN THE SKY [pun]
11 TEN+NISEL*+BOW
14 s/TABLE
15 TERMS [dd]
16 N[ECTAR*]INE

DOWN

2 MATTE/r
3 IN+CONTINENT
4 IRIS+H+SETTER
5 ANDES [hid]
6 HOT POTATO [pun]
7 KANYEWEST*
12 NO/ta/BLE
13 'BARON'

Puzzle 15 solution

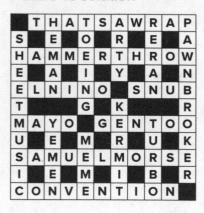

ACROSS

1 h/ARS/h+ENAL<
7 HALLUCINATE*
8 LOO+SEN
9 ISLE [alt]
11 'SIKH'
12 LETS GO [spoon]
14 MIDDLE-EARTH [reb]
15 PORT+RAY

DOWN

1 ALLWOR[K]EDUP*
2 SO+USED
3 N+OIR<
4 LEADS+f/AS/t+TRAY
5 W[HOLES]OME/n
6 BEHEMOTHS*
10 METEOR* [&lit]
13 SLUR [code]

Puzzle 16 solution

ACROSS

1 T[HAT+SAW]RAP
8 HAMMER+THROW
9 ELNINO*
10 SNUB<
12 MAY+O
14 GENT+OO
17 SAMUELMORSE*
18 CONVENTION [dd]

DOWN

2 HEM+AN
3 'TOEING'
4 p/ARTY
5 RERAN [hid]
6 PAWNBROKER [spoon]
7 SHEETMUSIC*
11 K+p/ERMIT
13 YEMEN*
15 TURB<+O
16 ME+ME

Puzzle 17 solution

D	A	T	U	M		B	A	B	E	L
U		A		O		R		U		U
G	O	B	A	L	L	I	S	T	I	C
		L		A		O		T		I
D	R	E	A	R	Y		B	E	E	F
E		T		S		G		R		E
F	L	E	X		C	O	F	F	E	R
I		N		O		T		L		
C	O	N	T	R	A	C	T	I	O	N
I		I		C		H		E		U
T	E	S	S	A		A	S	S	E	T

ACROSS

1 DA+TUM
4 BABE+L
7 GOBALLISTIC*
8 D[REAR]Y
9 B+E+E+F
11 'FLEX'
12 'COFFER'
14 CONTRACTION [dd]
16 TESSA<
17 AS+SET

DOWN

1 DUG [alt]
2 TABLET+ENNIS* [minus A]
3 MO+LARS
4 BRIO [man of BIRO]
5 B+UTTER+FLIES
6 LUCIFER*
8 'DEFICIT'
10 GOT[C]H+A
13 'ORCA'
15 NUT [dd]

Puzzle 18 solution

	S	A	T	I	S	F	I	E	D
	T		A		H		N		I
P	A	U	L	K	E	A	T	I	N	G
	N		O		E		R		N
	D	O	N	O	T	M	O	V	E
	O				A				R
	F	E	M	I	N	I	S	E	D
	F		A		C		I		R
B	I	L	L	Y	H	U	G	H	E	S
	S		T		O		N		S
	H	E	A	D	R	E	S	T	S

ACROSS

1 SAT+IS+F[I]ED
6 PAULK*+EATING
7 DONOTMOVE*
8 FE[MINIS]ED
11 BILLY+'HUGHES'
12 HEADRESTS*

DOWN

1 STAND+OF+FISH
2 T+s/ALON
3 'SHEE+TANCHOR'
4 INTRO* [minus AS]
5 DIN[NERD]RESS*
9 M[ALT]A
10 'SIGNS'

Puzzle 19 solution

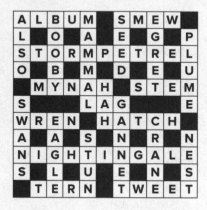

S	P	R	I	G		B	A	W	L	
A		H		E		A		E		A
P	R	O	C	L	A	I	M	I	N	G
S		D		A		L		G		O
	S	A	U	T	E		S	H	U	N
P			I	L	K					Y
L	O	B	E		L	I	S	L	E	
U		R		F		S		A		S
C	H	A	R	I	S	M	A	T	I	C
K		N		R		E		E		A
	E	D	A	M		T	E	X	A	N

DOWN
1 SAPS [dd]
2 RHODA*
3 GELATI [hid]
4 BAIL [dd]
5 'WEIGH'
6 AGO+NY
9 ELL [alt]
11 PLUCK [dd]
13 KISMET* [minus A]
15 BRAN+D
17 LATE+X
18 FIRM [man—R for L in FILM]
19 SC/otsm/AN

ACROSS
1 SPRI/n/G
4 'BAWL'
7 PROCLAIMING*
8 SAUTE [code]
10 S[H]UN
12 m/ILK
14 LOB+E
16 LISLE*
20 C[HARISMATI*]C
21 EDAM<
22 TEX/t+AN

Puzzle 20 solution

A	L	B	U	M		S	M	E	W	
L		O		A		E		G		P
S	T	O	R	M	P	E	T	R	E	L
O		B		M		D		E		U
	M	Y	N	A	H		S	T	E	M
S			L	A	G					E
W	R	E	N		H	A	T	C	H	
A		A		S		N		R		N
N	I	G	H	T	I	N	G	A	L	E
S		L		U		E		N		S
	T	E	R	N		T	W	E	E	T

DOWN
1 ALS+O
2 BOO+BY
3 M+'c/AMEL'
4 S/p/EED
5 EGRET< [hid]
6 PLUM+E
9 HAH [alt]
11 S[WAN]S [man—WAN for O in SOS]
13 GAN<+NET<
15 b/EAGLE
17 C+RANE*
18 ST+UN
19 NEST*

ACROSS
1 ALBUM [hid]
4 S[M]EW
7 STORMPETREL*
8 'MYNAH'
10 STEM [dd]
12 LAG [dd]
14 W/ar/REN
16 HATCH [code]
20 NIGH+TIN+GALE
21 'TERN'
22 TWEE+T

Puzzle 21 solution

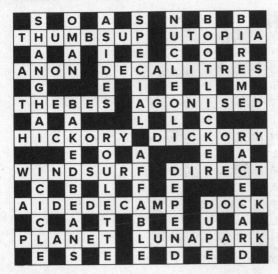

ACROSS

8 THUMBS+UP

9 U+TOPIA*

10 ANON [hid]

11 DECALITRES*

12 THE+BES/t

14 AGONISED*

15,17,24-ac HICK+OR+Y+
DICK+OR+Y+DOCK

20 WINDSURF* [FOURDOWNIS*
minus OO!]

22 DIRECT [dd]

23 AIDE*+DECAMP

25 PLA<+NET

26 LU[NAP+A]RK

DOWN

1 SHANGHAI [hid]

2 OM+AN

3 ASIDES [dd]

4 SPECIAL*

5 NUCLEOLI*

6 BOOT+'LICKER'

7 'BIREME'

13 BAKEDBEANS*

16 ROU[LET]TE

18 RACE CARD [dd]

19 A+F+FABLE

21 'b/ICICLE'

22 DE+PE+ND [code]

24 D[UP]E

Puzzle 22 solution

S	L	U	M	B	E	R		A	B	D	O	M	E	N
	E		A		G		N		O		N		R	
C	O	T	T	A	G	E	I	N	D	U	S	T	R	Y
	N		R		O		C		Y		E		A	
S	I	M	I	A	N		O	R	B	I	T	I	N	G
	N		A		T		U		L		D			
D	E	C	R	E	E	N	I	S	I		W	A	S	H
U		C		M		N		L		A				O
B	A	S	H		B	R	E	A	D	F	R	U	I	T
	I			E		P			E		N			
P	R	O	T	O	Z	O	A		T	A	H	I	T	I
	H		A		Z		T		A		O		E	
R	E	P	U	B	L	I	C	A	N	G	U	A	R	D
	A		N		E		H		K		S		I	
E	D	I	T	O	R	S		E	S	T	E	E	M	S

ACROSS

1 S+LUMBER
5 ABDOMEN*
10 COTTAGEINDUSTRY*
11 SI[MIA<]N
12 OR+BITING
13 DECREENIS*+I
15 W+ASH
17 BASH [dd]
19 'BREAD'+F[RU]IT
21 PROTOZOA*
23 TA+HIT+I
24 RE+PUBLICAN+GUARD*
25 EDITORS*
26 ESTEEMS< [hid]

DOWN

2 LE+O+NINE
3 MA[TRIA*]RCH
4 EGG ON [dd]
6 BODYBUILD*
7 ONSET [hid]
8 ER+RANDS
9 NICOTINEPATCH*
13 DUB [dd]
14 EMBEZZLER* [+ LMZ]
15 W[A]REHOUSE*
16 p/HOT/o
18 AI[RHEA]D
20 INTERIM [hid]
22 T+AUNT
23 TANKS [dd]

Puzzle 23 solution

D	E	P	A	R	T	S	■	T	H	E	A	T	R	E
Y	■	I	■	E	■	T	■	U	■	G	■	I	■	S
N	O	R	■	P	L	A	N	T	A	G	E	N	E	T
A	■	O	■	E	■	R	■	U	■	S	■	■	■	O
S	P	U	T	N	I	K	S	■	C	H	O	S	E	N
T	■	E	■	T	■	N	■	B	■	E	■	A	■	I
Y	E	T	I	■	C	A	S	A	B	L	A	N	C	A
■	■	T	■	C	■	K	■	B	■	L	■	C	■	■
P	R	I	V	A	T	E	E	Y	E	■	S	H	A	H
A	■	N	■	R	■	D	■	S	■	J	■	O	■	E
P	A	G	E	R	S	■	F	I	R	E	O	P	A	L
A	■	■	■	E	■	E	■	T	■	T	■	A	■	I
D	I	S	T	R	I	B	U	T	E	S	■	N	I	P
O	■	I	■	A	■	R	■	E	■	A	■	Z	■	A
C	H	R	I	S	T	O	■	R	A	M	R	A	I	D

ACROSS

1 D[EP]ARTS
5 THEATRE [dd]
9 'NOR'
10 PLANT+AGE+NET
11 S[PUT]NIKS<
12 CH+OSEN*
15 Y+ETI [alt]
16 CASA+BLANCA [dd—in Spanish!]
18 PRIVATE+EYE
19 SH+AH
22 PAGERS*
23 FIREOPAL*
25 DIS[T+RIB]UTES*
27 NIP [dd]
28 CHRISTO*
29 RAM[R]AID

DOWN

1 DY+NASTY
2 PI[ROUE]TTING
3 REPENT [pun]
4 STAR[K]NAKED*
5 'TU'+'TU'
6 EGGS+HE'LL
7 TIN/y
8 ESTONIA*
13 SANCHOP*+'ANZA'
14 BA/r+BY+SITTER
17 C+ARRERAS*
18 P[A+PAD]OC<
20 HE[LIP]AD
21 JETS+AM
24 EBRO< [hid]
26 SIR/i

Puzzle 24 solution

H	U	M	D	R	U	M		P	I	T	A	P	A	T
O		A		I		E		U		O		O		A
L	E	D		D	E	L	I	B	E	R	A	T	E	D
D		E		D		A		S		T				P
O	U	T	F	L	A	N	K		P	O	N	C	H	O
U		O		E		C		B		I		H		L
T	O	O	L		P	H	I	L	I	S	T	I	N	E
		R		C		O		A		E		C		
H	Y	D	R	A	U	L	I	C	S		S	K	I	T
A		E		N		Y		K		C		E		H
M	A	R	I	N	A		E	S	T	R	A	N	G	E
M			I		I		H		A		F		R	
O	K	T	O	B	E	R	F	E	S	T		E	G	O
C		O		A		A		E		E		E		U
K	R	E	M	L	I	N		P	A	R	A	D	O	X

ACROSS

1 HUM+DRUM
5 PITA+PAT
9 LED [dd]
10 DELIBERATED*
11 OUTFLANK*
12 PONCHO [hid]
15 TOOL<
16 'PHILISTINE'
18 HYDRAULICS*
19 SKIT/tles
22 MAR+IN+A
23 ESTRANGE*
25 OK+TO+BE+R[F]EST
27 EGO [hid]
28 KREMLIN [man—K for G in GREMLIN]
29 PARAD/e+OX

DOWN

1 HOLD OUT [dd]
2 MA[DETOOR<]DER*
3 RIDDLE [man – R for P in PIDDLE]
4 'MELANCHOLY'
5 PU<+BS
6 TORT+n/OISE
7 POT [dd]
8 TAD+POLE
13 CHICKEN FEED [dd]
14 BLACKSHEEP*
17 CAN+NIB+A+L
18 HAM+MOCK
20 T[HERO]UX
21 CRATER [pun]
24 I+RAN
26 TO+E

Puzzle 25 solution

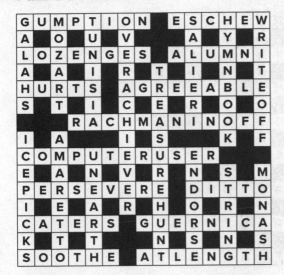

ACROSS

1 GUM+PTION*
5 ESCHEW [man—W for R in ESCHER]
9 LOZENGES [dd]
10 ALUMNI [hid]
12 'HURTS'
13 AGREEABLE*
14 RACHMAN*+IN-OFF
17 COMPUTERUSER*
22 PER[SEVER]E
23 DITTO< [hid]
24 CATE+RS
25 GUERNIC*+A
26 SOOT+HE
27 ATLENGTH*

DOWN

1 GAL<+AHS*
2 M[OZ]ART
3 TUNI*+a/SIA
4 OVERACHIEVER*
6 SA[LIE]RI
7 'HYMN'+BOOK
8 'WRITE OFF'
11 TREASUREHUNT*
15 ICE+PICKS
16 A+MARE[T]TO
18 UNEARTH [hid]
19 END+h/ORSE
20 STRING [dd]
21 M[ON]ASH

Puzzle 26 solution

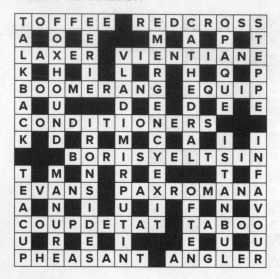

ACROSS

1 TO+F+FEE
4 RED+CROSS
9 LA[X]ER<
10 VIENTIANE*
11 BOOMERANG*
12 E+QUIP [pun]
13 CONDITION+ERS
17 BORISYELTSIN*
20 'EVANS'
21 PAXROMANA*
23 C+OUPDETAT*
24 TAB+OO
25 PHEASANT [hid]
26 ANG[L]ER

DOWN

1 TALKBACK [dd]
2 FOXHOUND [spoon]
3 E+ERIE
5 EMERGENCYEXIT*
6 CAT+HEDRAL*
7 OPAQUE [hid]
8 'STEPPE'
10 VLADI*+MIR<+PUT+IN
14 IRONSIDES*
15 IS+TAN+BUL/I
16 INFAVOUR*
18 TEACUP [code]
19 MANURE [pun]
22 OF+TEN

Puzzle 27 solution

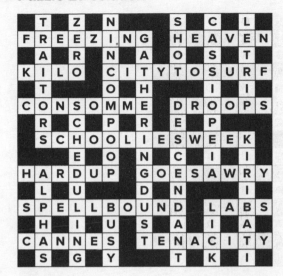

ACROSS

7 FREE+ZING
9 HEAVE+N
10 'KI'+'LO'
11 CITYTOSURF*
12 CONSOMME* [minus T]
14 DR+OOPS
15 SCHOOLIESWEEK*
17 HAR[DU]P
19 GO+ESAWRY*
20 SPELL+BOUND
22 LABS [dd]
23 C+ANNES
24 TEN+A+CITY

DOWN

1 TRAIT+w/ORS/t
2 ZERO [dd]
3 N+INCOM/e+POOP
4 SHOT [dd]
5 CASSIOPEIA*
6 LE+TRIP
8 GATHERING DUST [pun]
13 SCHEDULING* [minus I]
14 DESC[END]ANT
16 KIR+I[BAT]I
18 ALP+HAS
21 BUS+Y
22 LICK [dd]

Puzzle 28 solution

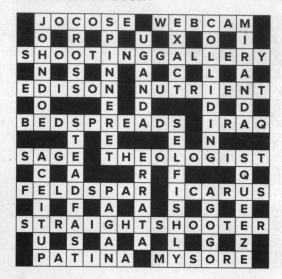

ACROSS

1 JO[CO]SE*
4 WE+B/e/CAM/e
9 SHOOTING+GALLERY
10 EDIS<+ON
11 NUT+RIENT*
12 BEDSPREADS [pun]
15 IRA+Q
16 SAGE [dd]
18 THEOLOGIST*
21 'FELD'+SPAR
23 ICARUS [pun]
25 STRAIGHT SHOOTER [pun]
26 PA+TINA
27 MY+SORE

DOWN

1 JOHN+DOE/s
2 CROSS [dd]
3 SP[INNER]ET
5 EX+ACT
6 COLLI/e+DING/o
7 MIR+AND+A
8 'U'+'GANDA'
13 STEADFAST*
14 SEL/I+FISH[L]Y
   [LACE 'discarded' = L]
17 ACEITUP*
19 ERRATA [hid]
20 SQUEEZE [dd]
22 P+AGA[i]N
24 AGOG+O

Puzzle 29 solution

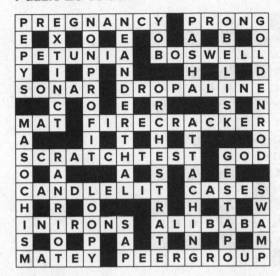

ACROSS

1 PREGNANCY [alt]
6 PRONG [man – P for W in WRONG]
9 PETUN[I]A*
10 BO+SWELL
11 SO+NAR<
12 DROP A LINE [pun]
14 MAT/ey
15 FIRE+CRACKER
17 SCRATCH+TEST
19 GOD [hid]
20 CANDLELIT*
22 CASES [dd]
24 IN IRONS [hid]
26 AL[I+BAB/y]A
27 MA+TEY<
28 PEER+GROUP

DOWN

1 'PEPYS'
2 t/EXT+IN+CT
3 NONPROFIT*
4 NEANDERTHAL*
5 YOB<
6 PASH+A
7 OBELISK*
8 GOLDENROD [pun]
13 'ORCHESTRATE'
14 M[ASOCHIS*]M
16 A+TT+ACHING
18 RANRIOT*
19 GESTAPO [hid]
21 LOOPY [pun]
23 SWA[M]P
25 SAP [dd]

Puzzle 30 solution

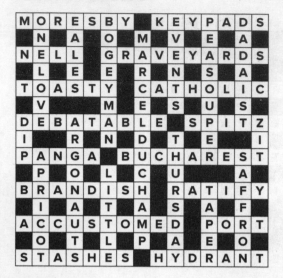

ACROSS

5 KEY+PADS
11 G+RAVEYARDS*
12 TO+A+STY
13 CATHOLIC*
14 DEBA*+TABLE
16 'SPITZ'
19 PANG+A
21 BU[CHARE*]ST
24 BRAN+DISH
25 g/RATIFY
27 ACCUS[TOM]ED
28,1 PORT+MORES+BY
29 ST+ASHES
30 HYDRANT*

DOWN

2 ONE LOVE [hid]
3 'EALES'
4 BOGEYMAN*
6 EVEN+TS
7 'PEA-SOUPER'
8 DAD+AIST*
9 MA+RCELDU*+CHAMP
14 DIP [dd]
15 'ARGO'+'NAUTS'
17 Z+IT
18 THURSDAY* [minus O]
20 APRI*+COT
22 S+AFFRON/t
23,10 LITTLE 'NELL' [pun]
26 TAPER [dd]

Puzzle 31 solution

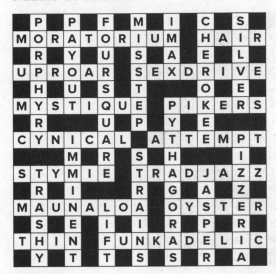

ACROSS

8 M[ORATOR+I]UM
9 HAIR [hid]
10 UPROAR* [minus AM]
11 SE[X]DRIVE*
12 MY+STIQUE*
13 PIKERS [dd]
14 CYNICAL*
16 AT+TEMPT
19 STYMIE*
21 TRA<+DJ+A+ZZ
23 'MAUNA'+'LOA'
25 OYSTER [hid]
26 THIN/g
27 FUNKADELIC*

DOWN

1 PORP<+HY+RY
2 PA+YOUT/h
3 FOUR-SQUARE/d
4 MISS+TEP<
5 cl/IMAX
6 C(HER)OKE+E
7 SILVER [dd]
13 PYTH/on+AGORAS
15 I+MM+IN/v/ENT
17 PIZ</ZERIA*
18 STRAINS [dd]
20 TRA[SH]Y
22 J+AS+PER
24 LI+FT (51 feet)

Puzzle 32 solution

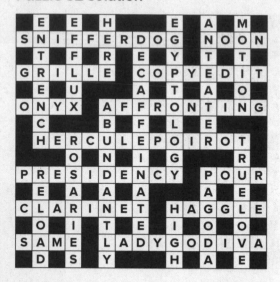

ACROSS

7   SNIFFERDOG* [+DS]
10 G[RILL]E
11 COPYEDIT* [minus ON]
12 ON-YX
13 AFFRONTING*
14 HERCULEPOIROT*
17 P+RESIDENCY
19 'POUR'
20 CLAR[IN]ET
21 HA[GG]LE
22,3 SAM+EH+ERE
23 LADY GODIVA [pun]

DOWN

1   g/ENT+'RENCH'
2   I/EF/t+FLU+X
4   EGYPTOLOGY [pun]
5   AN+TEAT+ER [alt]
6   MOTION [dd]
8   DECAFFE<+INATED*
13 ABUNDANTLY*
15 ROS/e+ARIES
16 TRUE+LOVE
18 RELOAD*
19 P.A.+'GODA'
21,9 HIGH NOON [pun]

Puzzle 33 solution

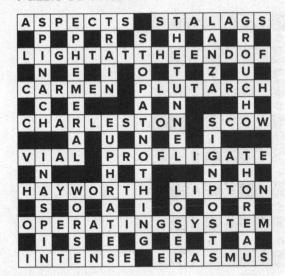

ACROSS

1   ASP+ECTS*
5   STALAGS*
10,6   LIGHT AT THE END OF THE TUNNEL [cryptic definition]
11   CAR+MEN
12   PLUT/o+ARCH
13   CHARLESTON*
15   S+COW
16   'VIAL'
18   PROFLIGATE*
20   HAY+WORTH
22   LIP+TON
23   OPERATINGSYSTEM*
24   IN+TENS+E
25   ERAS+MUS<

DOWN

2   S[PIN]ACH*
3   EP+H+EMERAL/d
4   TRAIN [dd]
7   LANZA [hid]
8   GROUCHO*
9   STOP AT NOTHING [pun]
14   'EUPH'+RATES
15   SIGN+POSTS
17   f/INA/l+SPIN<
19   THOR[E]AU* [&lit]
21   WOR<+SE
22   LOSER [dd]

Puzzle 34 solution

C		B	M			H		R		M	H
A	V	E	N	U	E		C	Y	R	A	N	O	D	E
R		R	S			P		T		D	B
D	O	G	L	E	G		M	E	N	S	W	E	A	R
I		E		U		P		R		T		R	E
G	A	R	A	M	M	A	S	A	L	A		N	E	W
A		A			R		C		I	
N	E	C	K	T	I	E		T	E	L	A	V	I	V
			I		N		I			E		I
R	O	B		N	A	T	I	V	E	T	I	T	L	E
I		E		T		H		E		O		E	T
P	R	I	M	A	T	E	S		R	U	B	R	I	C
O		R		C		S			R		A		O
F	A	U	L	K	N	E	R		L	E	A	N	O	N
F		T		S		S			D		S		G

ACROSS

8 A+VENUE [man – E for S in VENUS]
9,12 CYR*+ANODE+BERG+ERAC<
10 DOG+LEG
11 MENSWEAR*
13 GARAM*+'MASALA'
14 'NEW'
15 NECK+TIE
17 TELAV<+IV
20 ROB/e
22 NATIVETITLE*
24 PRIMATES [dd]
25 RUBRIC [hid]
26 FAUL[K]NER*
27 LE/b/ANON

DOWN

1 CARDI[GA]N
3 M[USE]UM
4 HYPERACTIVE*
5 RATS+'TAIL'
6,7 MODE+RN+HE+BREW
12 PARENT+HE'S+d/ES/k
16 TINTACKS*
18 VET+ERANS<
19 VIETCONG*
20 RIP-OFF [dd]
21 'BEIRUT'
23 TO+U+RED

Puzzle 35 solution

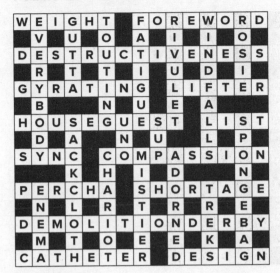

ACROSS

1,11 WEIGHTLIFTER*
5 FO<+REWORD [man − O for A in REWARD]
9 DESTRUCTIVENESS*
10 G[Y]RATING
12 HO[U+SEGUE]ST
16 LIST [dd]
18 'SYNC'
19 COMPASS+I+ON
24 S[HOR]TAGE
26 DEMOLITIONDERBY*
27 CA[THE]TER
28 DESIGN [hid]

DOWN

2 E+VERY+BODY*
3,22 'GUTTA'+'PERCHA'
4 T+OUTING
5 FAT+I+GUE/ss
6 RIV[UL]ET
7 WIND+FALLS
8 ROSI[alt]+E
13 S[ACKCLOT*]H
14 UNO [code]
15 SUP [dd]
17 SPONGE+BAG
19 C[HARI]OT
20 MIS[TI<]ER
21 A+'DORNED'
23 ENEMA< [hid]
25 'TREKS'

Puzzle 36 solution

D	E	C	O	R	U	M		J	A	V	E	L	I	N
O		O		U		A		O		I		O		O
S	T	R	I	D	E	N	C	Y		S	Q	U	A	W
A		P		O		I				I		T		A
G	H	O	U	L		P	R	A	C	T	I	S	E	D
E		R		P		B		O						A
	K	E	Y	H	O	L	E	S	U	R	G	E	R	Y
P		A			A		E			R				S
I	L	L	G	O	T	T	E	N	G	A	I	N	S	
N		N		E		T		E		M			A	
P	A	N	H	A	N	D	L	E		R	E	A	D	Y
O		Y		R		E		A		L			E	
I	G	L	O	O		S	C	I	N	T	I	L	L	A
N		O		L		A		S		E		E		Y
T	I	N	G	L	E	D		M	I	S	T	Y	P	E

ACROSS

1 DEC+O+RUM
5 JAV/a+ELIN<
9 STRIDENCY*
10 SQUA/d+W
11 e/G/o+s/HOUL/d
12 PRA[CT]ISED
14 KEYHOL[E]SURGERY*
17 ILL-GOTTEN GAINS [pun]
21 PAN-HANDLE [pun]
23 RE[AD]Y*
24 I+'GLOO'
25 SCINTILLA*
26 T+m/INGLED
27 MISTY+PE

DOWN

1 DO+SAGE
2 COR[PORE]AL
3 RU+DOLPH/in
4 e/M[ANIP*]ULATED
5 JOY [code]
6 VI+SITOR*
7 LOUTS [man – moving T in LOTUS]
8 NOWADAYS*
13 ABSENTEEISM* [+ BE]
15 ERNM*[alt]+ALLEY
16 PIN+POINT
18 ON A ROLL [pun]
19 AERATES* [minus W]
20 'AYE-AYE'
22 N+YLON*
25 SAD<

Puzzle 37 solution

N	A	S	H	I	P	E	A	R		S	Q	U	I	B

N	A	S	H	I	P	E	A	R	■	S	Q	U	I	B
O	■	P	■	S	■	C	■	O	■	A	■	S	■	O
V	I	E	W	S	■	H	E	M	A	N	D	H	A	W
A	■	C	■	U	■	I	■	P	■	G	■	E	■	W
K	N	I	F	E	E	D	G	E	■	F	E	R	M	I
■	■	A	■	■	N	■	R	■	R	■	■	■	■	N
P	O	L	E	N	T	A	■	S	C	O	F	F	E	D
E	■	F	■	I	■	■	■	■	I	■	O	■	O	■
T	A	X	I	C	A	B	■	J	U	D	E	L	A	W
R	■	■	A	■	Y	■	A	■	■	■	L	■	■	■
U	P	P	E	R	■	R	A	I	N	S	T	O	R	M
C	■	I	■	A	■	O	■	A	■	O	■	W	■	E
H	E	X	A	G	O	N	A	L	■	D	R	E	A	D
I	■	I	■	U	■	I	■	A	■	O	■	R	■	O
O	M	E	G	A	■	C	H	I	N	M	U	S	I	C

ACROSS

1 N[A+SHIP]EAR
6 SQUIB [dd]
9 VIE[W]S
10 HEMAN+DHA*+W
11 KNIFEEDGE*
12 FERMI< [hid]
13 POLE+NT+A
15 S[COFFE/e]D
17 TA[XI+CA]B
19 JUDE+LAW [spoon]
20 UPPER [dd]
22 b/RAINSTORM
25 HEX+AGONAL*
26 D[R]EAD
27 O+MEGA
28 CHI[NMUSI*]C

DOWN

1 NOV+A+K
2 SPECIALFX*
3 ISSUE [dd]
4 E[CHI]DNA
5 ROMPERS* [minus E]
6 SANGFROID*
7 p/USHER/s
8 BOWW[IN+D]OW
13 P+ETRUCHIO*
14 NICAR<+j/AGUA/r
16 FO/i/L+LOWERS
18 B+'YRONIC'
19 JAI[A]L+AI
21 P[IX]IE—or PI[XI]E
23 SOD+OM
24 ME+DOC

Puzzle 38 solution

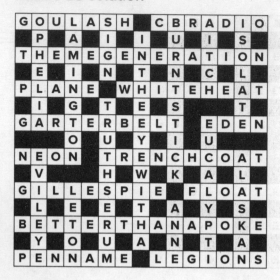

ACROSS

1 GOU/da+LASH
5 C[BRAD+I]O
10 THEME+GENERA+TION*
12 WHITEHEAT*
14 GARTERBELT* [minus Y]
15 E-DEN
16,4 NEON SIGN [spoon]
18 TRENCHCOAT*
20 GILL+ESPIE/d
22,11 FLOAT+'PLANE'
24,9,6 BETTER THAN A POKE IN
   THE EYE WITH A BURNT STICK
   [cryptic definition]
25 PENN[AM]E
26 LEGI/r/ONS

DOWN

2 OPHELIA*
3 LA+MING+TON
7 A+ITCH
8 ISO[alt]+LATE
13 TRUTHSE*+RUM
15 EUC<+ALY[P]TI*
17 EVILEYE* [+ EEE]
19 ALAS+'KAN'
21 L+ETON
23 ANNE [hid]

Puzzle 39 solution

R	E	G	I	C	I	D	E		S	T	A	D	I	A
I		O		O		I		B		O		N		N
P	A	P	A	L		C	H	E	C	K	M	A	T	E
P		A		U		E		R		Y		S		M
E	S	K	I	M	O	D	O	G		O	T	A	G	O
R			B			A				M				N
S	I	N	A	I		H	U	M	B	L	E	P	I	E
		I		N		O		O		O		L		
V	O	L	D	E	M	O	R	T		C	H	E	S	S
I		E		D				A						I
S	O	D	A	S		W	H	I	R	L	I	G	I	G
I		E		P		I		N		C		R		H
B	A	L	L	O	O	N	E	D		A	V	E	R	T
L		T		I		K		I		L		E		L
E	M	A	I	L	S		Z	E	A	L	O	T	R	Y

ACROSS

1 REG[ICI]DE
5 STADIA [hid]
10 PAPA+L
11 CHECK+MATE
12 ESKIMODOG*
13 O+TAG+O
14 'SINAI'
16 HUMBLE PIE [pun]
18 VOLDEMORT*
19 a/CHE+SS
21 SO+DAS
23 WHIRL+I+GIG
26 BALLOONED*
27 AVER+T
28 EM[A]ILS<
29 ZE+ALOT+RY

DOWN

1 RIPPERS [dd]
2 GO+'PAK'
3 COLUM/n+BIN+E
4 D+ICED
6 TO+KY+O
7 DNAS<+AMPLE
8 A+NEMO+NE
9 BERG+A+MOT
15 NILEDELTA*
16 HOO[DWIN*]K
17 LO-CAL+CALL
18 di/VISIBLE
20 S/I/IGHTLY
22 SP[O]IL<
24 INDI/cat/E
25 G/REET*

Puzzle 40 solution

A	P	O	L	O	G	Y		M	A	C	B	E	T	H
	H		O		R		R		L		E		H	
L	A	N	G	U	A	G	E	B	A	R	R	I	E	R
	L		I		S		I		C		N		A	
P	A	T	E	R	S	O	N		R	E	S	O	R	T
	N			Y		C		I		T		T		
E	X	I	S	T		P	A	S	T	T	E	N	S	E
			W		S		R		Y		I			
S	H	O	E	S	H	I	N	E		S	N	A	P	S
	O		A		E		A		I				R	
U	L	S	T	E	R		T	I	M	E	P	O	O	R
	S		S		I		I		P		S		S	
A	T	T	H	E	D	R	O	P	O	F	A	H	A	T
	E		O		A		N		R		L		I	
P	R	O	P	A	N	E		S	T	O	M	A	C	H

ACROSS

1 A+POLO+G/u/Y
5 MACBETH [pun]
10 LANGU[AGE]BARRIER*
11 PATERSON*
12 RESORT [dd]
13 s/EXIST/s
15 PAST+TENSE
17 SHOESHINE [pun]
19 SNAPS [dd]
22 'ULSTER'
23 TIMEPOOR*
25 AT THE DROP OF A HAT
    [MA/hat/MA = MAMA]
26 PROP[A+N]E/r
27 STOMACH [dd]

DOWN

2 PHALA*+NX [alt]
3 LOG[I]E
4 GRASSY [man—R for L in GLASSY]
6 A-LA+C[R]ITY
7 BERN+STEIN
8 T+HEARTS
9 RE/d+IN+CARNATION
14 SWEATSHOP*
16 SHERIDAN [hid]
18 HOLSTER [pun]
20 P+ROSAIC*
21 IMPORT [dd]
24 P[S]ALM

Puzzle 41 solution

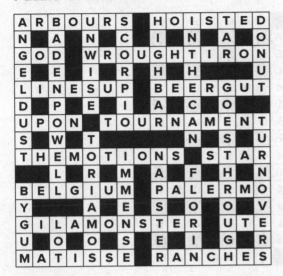

ACROSS

1 h/ARBOURS
5 HOISTED* [minus N]
9 GO+D
10 'WROUGHT'+IRON
11 LINES UP [dd]
12 BEER GUT [pun]
14 U[PO]N
15 T[OUR+NAME]NT
21 STAR [dd]
23 B[EL+GI]UM
24 PALER+MO
25 GILAMONSTER*
27 UTE [dd]
28 M[A+T]ISSE/s
29 b/RANCHES

DOWN

1 ANGELDUST*
2 BA[DEN+POWE/r]LL
3 UN[W]IS+E
4 SCOR/e+PI+O
5 HIGH+BAR
6 INTHECAN* [mixing NINTHACE]
7 s/TAR
8 DO+NUT
13,18 GOES THROUGH THE
MOTIONS [pun]
16 T[URN]OVERS*
17 TORIAMOS*
19 IM[MEN]SE
20 NAPSTER< [hid]
22 FLORIN* [minus L and S]
23 BY GUM [pun]
26 LOT [dd]

Puzzle 42 solution

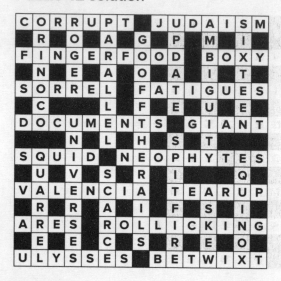

ACROSS

1 CO[RRUP<]T
5 JU[DAIS]M/p
10 FINGERFO*+OD<
11 BO[X]Y
12 SO[RR]EL*
13 FATIGUES [dd]
14 DOCUMENTS*
16,18 GIANTS[man]+QUID
   [I for R in GRANTS]
20 NEO*+'PHYTES'
23 VA[LE]N+CIA
24 T[EAR]UP<
26 ARES [alt]
27 ROLL+n/ICKING
28 ULYSSES [hid]
29 BE[TWIX]T

DOWN

2 O+RINO*+CO
3 ROGER [dd]
4,15 PARALLEL UNIVERSES [reb]
6 UP+DATE
7 AM[BIG+U]ITY
8 SIXTEEN* [minus CE]
9 GOOF+FTHERAILS*
17 SPIT<+FIRE
19 QUARREL [dd]
21 EQUIN/e+OX
22 SCARCE*
25 ASK+EW<

Puzzle 43 solution

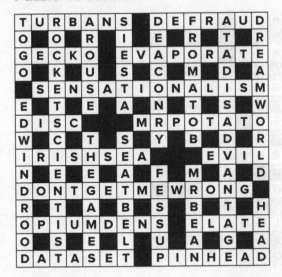

ACROSS

1 TURB<+ANS [alt]
5 D/e/E[FRAU]D
9 G+'ECKO'
10 EVAP<+ORATE
11 SENSATIONALISM*
13 DISC/over
14,22 MRPOTATOHEAD*
17 IRISH SEA [pun]
18 EVIL [hid]
21 DONTGETMEWRONG*
23 OPIUMD[E]NS*
24 ELATE [code]
25 DA+TASET*
26 PINHEAD [pun]

DOWN

1,6 TOGO+FROMATOB*
2 ROCKETSCIENTIST*
3 A+R[O]USE
4 SIESTA [hid]
5 DEACONRY*
7 ATADISADVANTAGE*
[DATA+DATA+VEGANIS]
8 DREAM*+'WORLD'
12 ED+WIND+ROOD<
15 TH[EG]AMES
16 SEAT+BELT
19 FE+SSUP<
20 MR BEAN [pun]

Puzzle 44 solution

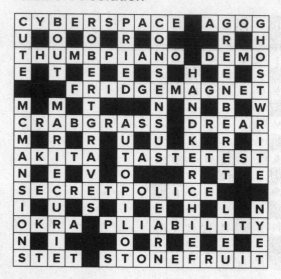

ACROSS

1 CYBERSPACE*
6 AGOG [hid]
9 THUMBPIANO*
10 DE+MO
12 FRIDGEMAG*+NET
15 CR[ABGR*]ASS
17 DR+EAR [pun]
18 A+KIT/e+A
19 TASTE+TEST
20 SECRETPOLICE*
24 O+KRA<
25 P+LIABILITY
26 STET/son
27 STONEFRUI*+T

DOWN

1 CUT-E
2 a/BOUT
3 f/RO/m+BE['RT']G+RAVES
4 'PRIED'
5 CON+'SENSUS'
7 GREE[NB+ERE]T
8 'GHOS'+'TWRITE'
11 HAND+KER/b+CHIEF
13 MCM+ANSIONS* [minus DT]
14 MAR[I]E+CUR[I]E
16 A+UT[alt]+OPILOT*
21 LEAR+N/ash
22 LIEU/tenant
23 N+YET

Puzzle 45 solution

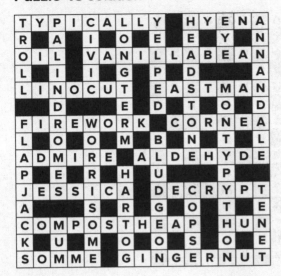

ACROSS

1 TYPICALLY [man − Y for O in TOPICALLY]
6 HYENA [hid]
9 OIL [dd]
10 VANILLABEAN* [+ NN]
11 LI+NOCUT*
12 EAST+MAN
14 FIRE+WORK
16 CORN+EA/r
18 AD+MIRE
19 ALDE*+HYDE
21 J+ESSICA*
22 DEC+'RYPT'
25 COMPOSTHEAP*
27 HUN/t
28 SOMME< [hid]
29 GINGER NUT [pun]

DOWN

1 TROLL [dd]
2 PALIN+D+ROMES
3 CIVIC [Roman numerals]
4 LONG-TERM [pun]
5 YELPED*
6 HEADSTONE [pun]
7 EYE [dd]
8 A+N/u/N+AND+ALE
13 MON[TYP/icall/Y]TH+ON
14 FLAP+JACKS
15 WOR<+RISOME*
17 BLUDGE+ON
20 'HART'+OG<
23 'COPSE'
24 TENET [palindrome]
26 MUM [versus MOM]

Puzzle 46 solution

	S	M	G	C		H		F		A	
P	A	R	A	G	U	A	Y		I	S	R	A	E	L
	L	L	I	P		G		O		G	
F	I	J	I		N	O	R	T	H	K	O	R	E	A
	N		E	E		B		T		A	
U	G	A	N	D	A		S	C	O	T	L	A	N	D
	E		O		S		R		O	
E	R	I	T	R	E	A		A	N	D	O	R	R	A
	T		M		M				P		A	
E	T	H	I	O	P	I	A		R	U	S	S	I	A
	E		N		H		J		E		N	
B	A	N	G	L	A	D	E	S	H		C	U	B	A
	B		H		S		S		E		O		A	
M	A	L	A	W	I		T	H	A	I	L	A	N	D
	G		M		S		Y		T		T		D	

ACROSS

8 PAR[A]GU[A]Y
9 IS+RAEL<
10 FIJ<+I
11 NORTH[KO+R]EA*
12 UGANDA [hid]
14 S[COTL*]AND
15 ERITREA* [minus S]
17 'ANDORRA'
20 g/ET/s+t/HI/s+c/OP/y+b/IA/s
22 'RUSSIA'
23 BANG+LADESH*
24 s/CUBA
25 M[A+LAW]I
26 T+HA[ILA<]ND

DOWN

1 SALI[NG]ER*
2 MAL/aw/l
3 GUINEA [dd]
4 'CYPRESS'
5 HIGH-BORN [spoon]
6 FROOTLOOPS*
7 'AEGEAN'
13 NOTTINGHAM [pun]
16 EMPHASIS*
18 RAINB*+AND
19 M[A+JEST]Y
21 TE[A+BA]G< [GET-up]
22 REHEAT*
24 COL+T

Puzzle 47 solution

A	C	R	O	P	O	L	I	S		Q	U	A	I	L
P		O		R		U		A		U		T		O
A	R	O	S	E		T	I	M	W	I	N	T	O	N
T		S		V		E		P		C		O		E
H	A	T	T	I	E		B	I	C	K	E	R	E	R
E				E		L		C				N		
T	E	D		W	E	E	D	K	I	L	L	E	R	S
I		R		E		S		L		I		Y		N
C	L	O	U	D	S	T	R	E	E	T		S	K	I
		P				E		S		T				V
R	A	S	P	F	E	R	N		E	L	A	I	N	E
O		I		I		L		C		E		L		L
B	A	C	K	S	L	A	S	H		O	R	I	E	L
E		A		H		M		U		W		A		E
D	O	L	L	Y		B	U	B	B	L	E	C	A	R

ACROSS

1 A+CROP+OLIS<
6 QU[A]IL/I
9 A+ROSE
10 TIM[WINT/er]ON
11 HAT[alt]+TIE
12 BICKERER* [minus EA]
14 TED* [minus CRUELSOT]
16 WEEDKILLERS*
19 CLOU[DSTREE*]T
20 SKI [dd]
21 RAS[P]FERN*
23 ELAINE< [hid]
26 BACKS/LASH
27 OR/f/IEL/d
28 DOLLY [man—O for A in DALLY]
29 BUBBLECAR* [ACRUEL + BBB]

DOWN

1 APATHETIC [hid]
2 ROOST*
3 P/REVIEWED
4 k/LUTE
5 S[AMP]ICKLES
6 QUICK [dd]
7 AT+TO/u/RNEYS
8 LON+ER [more like Lon]
13 L[ESTER*]LAM<+B
15 DROPSICAL*
17 LITTLEOWL* [+ LL]
18 S[NIV<]ELLER
21 R[OB]ED
22 FISH-Y
24 ILI+AC
25 CHUB [dd]

Puzzle 48 solution

	M	G	U	S	E	D	S						
L	A	C	R	O	S	S	E		S	H	I	N	T	Y
	J	A		A	A	C	R		U
G	O	L	F		G	Y	M	N	A	S	T	I	C	S
	R		E		I		P		Y		C
D	I	S	C	U	S		L	E	A	P	F	R	O	G
	T		A		E		D		A
C	Y	C	L	I	N	G		F	E	N	C	I	N	G
	E		E		C			E		O
H	A	N	D	B	A	L	L		C	A	S	I	N	O
	R		O		T		O		E		A
L	A	W	N	T	E	N	N	I	S		L	U	G	E
	F		I		N		I		S		O		O
K	A	R	A	T	E		N	I	N	E	P	I	N	S
	T		N		D		G		A		E		S

ACROSS

8 L+A+CROSS+E
9 SHIN[T]Y
10 GOLF<
11 GYMNASTICS [alt]
12 DISCUS/s
14 LEAPFROG* [GRAF + LOPE]
15 CY/CLING
17 FENCING [triple meaning]
20 HANDBALL [spoon]
22 CAS/h+IN+O
23 LAWNTENNIS*
24 LU/n/GE
25 K+A+RATE
26 NINE+PINS

DOWN

1 MAJ<+f/OR+c/ITY
2 GRAF/t
3 sa/USAGES
4 SEAMILE*
5 ES/C[A+PAD]E
6 DIRTY+F+ACES
7 STUCCO* [minus AN]
13 CALEDONIAN*
16 NE[A+TEN]ED [in NEED]
18 NONA+GONS<
19 CL+'ONING'
21 A+RAF[A]T
22 CESSNA< [hid]
24 LOP+E

Puzzle 49 solution

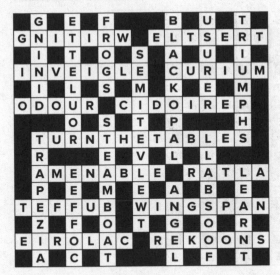

ALL 'TABLE' ANSWERS ARE TURNED AS PER THE CENTRAL PHRASE.

ACROSS

7 WRITING
[man – R for A in WAITING]
8 TRESTLE*
10 INVEIGLE*
11 CU+R[I]UM
12 O+DOUR
13 PERIODIC< [hid]
15 TURNTHETABLES*
17 A[MEN]A+BL/u/E
19 s/ALT+b/AR/k
22 BUFFET [dd]
23 WINGSPAN*
24 CALORIE [hid]
25 SNOOKER [pun]

DOWN

1 D/iv/INING
2 'ROULETTE'
3 FROGS [code]
4 BLACKOPA*+L
5 s/U/m+SURER
6 TRI[UMP]HS*
9 TW[EL+VET+IM]ES*
14 S[TEAM+BOA]T
15 TRAP+EZIA/b/<
16 FOOSBALL*
18 'COFFEE'
20 LE[AR]NT
21 ANGEL [man—L for R in ANGER]

Puzzle 50 solution

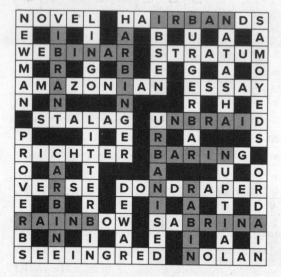

STARRED ANSWERS OMIT THEIR REWORDED 'BRAIN' ELEMENTS, FULLY REVEALED ABOVE.

ACROSS

1 NO[V]EL
*4 H+ADS
*9 WE
10 STRAT<+UM
11 AMAZ/e+ON+I+b/AN/k
12 t/ES/t+SAY [&lit]
13 STAL/e+AG/e
*15 UD [code]
17 RICH[T]ER
*19 G
22 VERSE [dd]
23 DONDRAPER* [&lit]
*25 OW
*26 'SA'
27 SEEINGRED* [minus S]
28 NOLAN< [alt]

DOWN

1 NEW+MAN
*2 VT<
3 LIN<+GO
*4 H[u]GER
5 n/IBS+EN
6 BURGERBAR* [&lit]
7 NAT+A<+SH+A
8 SAMOYEDS*
14 LIT+TER[BI]N
*15 USED
16 PRO+VERBS
*18 CE
20 NUPTIAL*
21 OR+'DAIN'
23 DE-WAR [pun]
24 [no scope for wordplay!]

ACKNOWLEDGEMENTS

Entering the brain is no easy thing. Despite the fact our skulls cradle the organ all day, so close we might touch it, the mystic pulp seems exiled to another dimension.

Even if you were to spy on the brain in a lab, what would you learn? Where would you even start? Its lobes are too complex, too vulnerable, to accommodate curious amateurs, and the wave-like graphs arising from clinical trials read as an alien language.

Hence this amateur needed brainy people in his corner, the insiders of this inner space, to illuminate the cavern we carry above, to unpack the cave's delicate contents. For this book to exist, I needed the fMRI firm on my autodial, a host of neural angels to translate gyri and sulci, the basal ganglia and the somatosensory cortex, to explain how thoughts emerge and shuttle.

The first such angel came out of the blue, the newest neurologist in Melbourne, Sarah Holper. Just when every research paper seemed a foreign document, when every clinic I'd pestered was courteous but not collaborative, a neurologist-in-training sent me an email, unsolicited. Sarah was then a relative pup in the field of brain research, an intern yet to qualify as doctor. She wished to talk about crosswords while I wished to talk about brains. Together, the gist of those chats proved to be this book's genesis, as well as the pilot study that saw a periscope crown my nose.

Far more than a sounding board, Dr Holper (as she made the grade mid-manuscript) has been my guide in a strange domain, a door opener, a catalyst, an interpreter, shedding light on the cerebellum's workings as much as how research trials are initiated, and how they operate.

Indeed, in the Florey's aftermath, my brain meeting some 300 clues in a tube, the results are still being cross-examined and calibrated, over a year since the experiment. (Keep in mind the study was a professional act of curiosity, a revolutionary bout of nosiness rather than a flagship project attracting full funding.) Of course, even with the luxury of funded hours, the cryptic trial would still retain a cryptic dimension in some part, owing to the multi-level puzzle the data generated. Not just a brain at rest, mine was a mind in full flight, juggling letters, unpacking puns and double-stepping homophones. Add to this the sprawl of brain actions, the intricacy of time splintered down into scans-per-second, the clues' spread of difficulty and their type, the occasional false answer, or the knock-on effect of a missed answer, and you start to grasp how a complete report may yet be a stretch away. Though there's no doubting the team's resolve to see where this world-first probe may lead. To that end, I can only trust my role as patient zero, on top of this book's mental adventure, will contribute to the ultimate aha.

For their part in Operation Cryptic, I'm indebted to the trio at the Florey Institute of Neuroscience and Mental Health, namely Dr Holper and her senior colleagues, Associate Professor David Abbott and cognitive neurologist Associate Professor David Darby.

Rousing cheers also for Professor Jennie Ponsford, the director of the Monash-Epworth Rehabilitation Research Centre, and speech pathologist Jennifer Brown at the Macquarie University Hospital—two more gatekeepers who were game—or foolhardy enough—to consider scanning a solver's brain at play. Thanks also to neuropsychologist Maggie Phillips, who floated the possibility of a puzzle trial in the first place, an idle remark she let slip on an afternoon bush walk.

To my friends at Dementia Australia, including Maree McCabe, Dr Kaele Stokes, Neil Samuel and Christine Bolt: you have been ferocious advocates. As my own dad eventually succumbed to frontal lobe dementia in 2013, I've been a proud ambassador for the cause, and I appreciate your contributions to this project, in offering both manuscript advice as well as the latest research findings.

Which seems my cue to cross to the beloved elders at the University of the Third Age, the crossword tribe who defy all talk of cognitive decline, meeting every second week to wrangle deceptions. You inspire us all.

I'd also like to thank Neo for his malingering confessions, as recorded in the *Together* chapter. As both a coder (and lunchtime decoder), Neo must retain his alias to deflect any accusations that his workplace puzzle-cracking is more important than, well, work.

Warm applause for Dr Debra Aarons, who lectures in linguistics at the University of New South Wales. Patient to the nth, Debra had the stamina to dismantle Chomskyian algorithms across a genial exchange of emails, the better to frame her research into playful clue-conquering. If colourless green ideas sleep furiously, then they do so under Debra's caring eye.

Overseas, the Buckingham investigators—doctors Kathryn Friedlander and Philip Fine—have offered no less vigorous assistance, delving deep into their research of the puzzle-solving elite. I look forward to seeing the same pair extend our understanding of crosswords as a benign addiction, from Bangalore to Singapore. And please, count me in. The world can never learn enough about how puzzling keeps us thriving.

Crossword setters from across the United Kingdom and the United States also need saluting, the legion of magicians whose sample clues adorn the book's second part. While a byline sits beside each clue, crediting the setters from Arachne to Vlad, I'd like to add my appreciation of your mind-bending here. Via your weekly Qaos, you spare a million brains from the Mudd, and I'm as grateful as any other solver.

Last in line are the book-dreamers at Allen & Unwin, where publisher Jane Palfreyman saw the sense of entering the brain in the first place, while the editorial A-team of Angela Handley, Ali Lavau and Aziza Kuypers has been dynamic in solving the manuscript's own mental challenges, not least the arrangement of sections, sentences, cubes and matchsticks.

Did I say last? My brain must be lapsing. I'd like to thank Tracy O'Shaughnessy for her constant support and insight, both within and beyond these covers. There's a chance our next coffee might dodge any talk of brains or clues, but it's a slim one.

Which reminds me. The sooner I wrap these acknowledgements, the quicker I can pounce on my next puzzle to untangle. Wish me luck—and may your own brain bloom in search of its own ahas.

REFERENCES

The Experiment

Kovach, Christopher K., Nathaniel D. Daw, David Rudrauf, Daniel Tranel, John P. O'Doherty and Ralph Adolphs, 'Anterior prefrontal cortex contributes to action selection through tracking of recent reward trends', *Journal of Neuroscience*, 20 June 2012, vol. 32, no. 25, pp. 8434–42

Introduction

Greenfield, Susan, *The Human Brain: A guided tour*, London: Weidenfeld & Nicolson, 1997

Let the brain tour begin

Geschwind, Norman and Walter Levitsky, 'Human Brain: Left–right asymmetries in temporal speech region', *Science*, 12 July 1968, vol. 161, issue 3837, pp. 186–7

Grandin, Temple, *Animals Make Us Human: Creating the best life for animals*, Boston: Mariner Books, Houghton Mifflin Harcourt, 2009

Layton, Julia, 'How does the body make electricity—and how does it use it?' HowStuffWorks, <https://health.howstuffworks.com/human-body/systems/nervous-system/human-body-make-electricity.htm>, accessed 6 May 2018

Aha—*The euphoria of eureka*

Sheth, Bhavin R., Simone Sandkühler and Joydeep Bhattacharya, 'Posterior Beta and Anterior Gamma Oscillations Predict Cognitive Insight', *Journal of Cognitive Neuroscience*, July 2009, vol. 21, issue 7, pp. 1269–79

Limb, Charles, 'Your brain on improv', [video] *TEDxMidAtlantic*, November 2010, <www.ted.com/talks/charles_limb_your_brain_on_improv>, accessed 6 May 2018

Tempo—*Pouncing versus pacing*

Kounios, John and Mark Beeman, 'The Aha! Moment: The cognitive neuroscience of insight', *Current Directions in Psychological Science*, 2009, vol. 18, no. 4, pp. 210–16

Kahneman, Daniel, *Thinking, Fast and Slow*, New York: Farrar, Straus and Giroux, 2011

Alter, Adam, Nicholas Epley, Rebecca Eyre and Daniel Oppenheimer, 'Overcoming Intuition: Metacognitive Difficulty Activates Analytic Reasoning', *Journal of Experimental Psychology*, 2007, vol. 136, no. 4, pp. 569–76

Focus—*The endangered art of being present*

Hutchison, RM and JB Morton, 'Tracking the Brain's Functional Coupling Dynamics over Development', *The Journal of Neuroscience*, 29 April 2015, vol. 35, issue 17, pp. 6849–59

Sullivan, Bob and Hugh Thompson, 'Brain, Interrupted', *The New York Times, Sunday Review*, 3 May 2013, <www.nytimes.com/2013/05/05/opinion/sunday/a-focus-on-distraction.html>, accessed 6 May 2018

The Norwegian University of Science and Technology (NTNU), 'Brain waves and meditation', *ScienceDaily*, <www.sciencedaily.com/releases/2010/03/100319210631.htm>, accessed 6 May 2018

Danesi, Marcel, *The Puzzle Instinct: The meaning of puzzles in human life*, Bloomington: Indiana University Press, 2004

Holloway, Jeffrey, *Mindfulness for Beginners: A simple, concise and complete guide to mindfulness meditation*, CreateSpace Independent Publishing Platform, 2017

Memory—*Your brain as active archive*

Skotko, Brian, Elizabeth Kensinger, Joseph Locascio, Gillian Einstein, David Rubin, Larry Tupler, Anna Krendl and Suzanne Corkin, 'Puzzling Thoughts for H.M.: Can new semantic information be anchored to old semantic memories?', *Neuropsychology*, 2004, vol. 18, no. 4, pp. 756–69

Jebelli, Joseph, *In Pursuit of Memory: The fight against Alzheimer's*, London: John Murray, 2018

Lennox, Graham and Iain Wilkinson, *Essential Neurology*, 4th edition, Hoboken: Wiley-Blackwell, 2005

Wesnes, Keith, 'The relationship between the frequency of word puzzle use and cognitive function in a large sample of adults aged 50 to 96 years', University of Exeter, 17 July 2017, <www.exeter.ac.uk/news/featurednews/title_595009_en.html>

Landau, Susan, Shawn Marks, Elizabeth Mormino, Gil Rabinovici, Hwamee Oh, James O'Neil, Robert Wilson and William Jagust, 'Association of lifetime cognitive engagement and low ß-amyloid deposition', *Archives of Neurology*, May 2012, vol. 69, issue 5, pp. 623–9

Kelly, Lynne, *The Memory Code*, Crows Nest: Allen & Unwin, 2016

Hirst, Graeme, Regina Jokel, Ian Lancashire and Xuan Le, 'Longitudinal detection of dementia through lexical and syntactic changes in writing: a case study of three British novelists', *Literary and Linguistic Computing*, vol. 26, issue 4, 1 December 2011, pp. 435–61

Dementia Australia, <www.dementia.org.au>

Vocabulary—*How porous is your thesaurus?*

United Nations World Food Programme, <www.freerice.com>

For more on Erin Barker of The Moth fame, see <https://themoth.org/storytellers/erin-barker>

Huth, Alexander, Wendy de Heer, Thomas Griffiths, Frédéric Theunissen and Jack Gallant, 'Natural speech reveals the semantic maps that tile human cerebral cortex', *Nature*, 28 April 2016, vol. 532, issue 7600, pp. 453–8

Haha—*Hip-hip for the hippocampus*

For more on Christine Hooker's research, see Amy Lavoie, 'It's all in the cortex', *Harvard Gazette*, March 2010

Schott, Ben, *Schottenfreude: German words for the human condition*, New York: Blue Rider Press, 2013

Play—*Survival of the funnest*

Kane, Pat, *The Play Ethic*, London: Pan Macmillan, 2004

Friedlander, Kathryn and Philip Fine, 'The grounded expertise components approach in the novel area of cryptic crossword solving', *Frontiers in Psychology*, May 2016, vol. 7, pp. 1–21

Dis/connect—*Time to break and remake*

Pullum, Geoffrey, 'Beware the Misles', *Lingua Franca*, Chronicle of
    Higher Education, 1 December 2011, <www.chronicle.com/blogs/
    linguafranca/2011/12/01/beware-the-misles/> accessed 6 May 2018

Johnson, Steven, *Where Good Ideas Come From*, New York: Riverhead, 2010

Herculano-Houzel, Suzana, 'What is so special about the human brain?' [video]
    TedGlobal, June 2013, <www.ted.com/talks/suzana_herculano_houzel_
    what_is_so_special_about_the_human_brain>, accessed 6 May 2018

Aarons, Debra, 'Following orders: Playing fast and loose with language and
    letters', *Australian Journal of Linguistics*, 2015, vol. 35, pp. 351–80

Together—*Thinking in harmony*

James, Bryan, Robert Wilson, Lisa Barnes and David Bennett, 'Late-life
    social activity and cognitive decline in old age', *Journal of International
    Neuropsychology Society*, November 2011, vol. 17, issue 6, pp. 998–1005

Surowiecki, James, *The Wisdom of Crowds*, New York: Little, Brown, 2004

University of the Third Age, <www.u3a.org.au>

Showtime

Scholz, Jan, Miriam Klein, Timothy Behrens and Heidi Johansen-Berg,
    'Training induces changes in white-matter architecture', *Nature
    Neuroscience*, 2009, vol. 12, issue 11, pp. 1370–1, <www.nature.com/
    articles/nn.2412>

SELECTED BIBLIOGRAPHY

Aamodt, Sandra and Sam Wang, *Welcome to Your Brain: Why you lose your car keys but never forget how to drive and other puzzles of everyday life*, London: Bloomsbury, 2008

Alter, Adam, *Drunk Tank Pink: The subconscious forces that shape how we think, feel and behave*, London: Oneworld, 2013

Brockman, John (ed.), *Thinking: The new science of decision-making, problem-solving and prediction*, New York: Harper Perennial, 2013

Corballis, Michael, *Pieces of Mind: 21 short walks around the human brain*, Melbourne: Scribe Publications, 2012

Danesi, Marcel, *The Puzzle Instinct: The meaning of puzzles in human life*, Bloomington: Indiana University Press, 2004

de Bono, Edward, *Six Thinking Hats*, London: Penguin, 2008

Doidge, Norman, *The Brain That Changes Itself* (revised edition), Melbourne: Scribe Publications, 2008

Eagleman, David, *Incognito: The secret lives of the brain*, Edinburgh: Canongate Books, 2011

——*The Brain: The story of you*, Edinburgh: Canongate Books, 2015

Eastaway, Rob, *Secrets of Lateral Thinking: 101 ideas for thinking creatively*, New York: Shelter Harbor Press, 2016

Fine, Cordelia (introduction), *The Britannica Guide to the Brain: A guided tour of the brain—Mind, memory, and intelligence*, London: Robinson, 2008

Gazzaniga, Michael S, *Tales from Both Sides of the Brain: A life in neuroscience*, New York: Ecco, 2015

Gibb, Barry J, *The Rough Guide to the Brain*, London: Rough Guides, 2007

Greenfield, Susan, *The Human Brain: A guided tour*, London: Weidenfeld & Nicolson, 1997

Jebelli, Joseph, *In Pursuit of Memory: The fight against Alzheimer's*, London: John Murray, 2018

Johnson, Steven, *Where Good Ideas Come From: The natural history of innovation*, New York: Riverhead Books, 2010

Kahneman, Daniel, *Thinking, Fast and Slow*, New York: Farrar, Straus and Giroux, 2011

Kelly, Lynne, *The Memory Code*, Sydney: Allen & Unwin, 2016

Knight, Eric, *Reframe: How to solve the world's trickiest problems*, Melbourne: Black Inc, 2012

Medina, John, *Brain Rules: 12 principles for surviving and thriving at work, home and school*, Melbourne: Scribe Publications, 2011

——*Brain Rules for Ageing Well: 10 principles for staying vital, happy and sharp*, Melbourne: Scribe Publications, 2018

New Scientist, *How Your Brain Works: Inside the most complicated object in the universe*, London: John Murray Learning, 2017

Restak, Richard, *The Playful Brain: The surprising science of how puzzles improve the mind*, New York: Riverhead Books, 2010

Robison, John Elder, *Switched On: A memoir of brain change, emotional awakening and the emerging science of neurostimulation*, New York: Spiegel & Grau, 2016

Rock, David, *Your Brain at Work: Strategies for overcoming distraction, regaining focus, and working smarter all day long*, London: Harper Collins, 2009

Rose, Steven, *The 21st-Century Brain: Explaining, mending and manipulating the mind*, London: Jonathan Cape, 2005

Sims, Peter, *Little Bets: How breakthrough ideas emerge from small discoveries*, New York: Free Press, 2011

Swaab, Dick, *We Are Our Brains: From the womb to Alzheimer's*, London: Allen Lane, 2014

Vogel, Thomas, *Breakthrough Thinking: A guide to creative thinking and idea generation*, New York: How Books, 2014

Wilkinson, Iain and Graham Lennox, *Essential Neurology*, 4th edition, Hoboken: Wiley-Blackwell, 2005

Wiseman, Richard, *59 Seconds: Think a little, change a lot*, London: Macmillan, 2009